Anti Inflammatory Diet

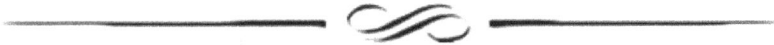

A 30 Day Meal Plan to Reduce Inflammation and Heal Your Body with Simple, fast, delicious and Healthy Recipes

Emily Hudson

The content within this book has been derived from various sources. Please consult a licensed professional before attempting any techniques outlined in this book.

By reading this document, the reader agrees that under no circumstances is the author responsible for any losses, direct or indirect, that are incurred as a result of the use of the information contained within this document, including, but not limited to, errors, omissions, or inaccuracies.

Table of Contents

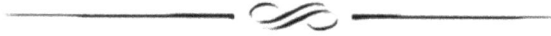

Introduction

Inflammation is a natural process with the biological purpose to initiate healing by increasing circulation. It is a complex process involving both the immune system and vascular system and the interplay of various chemical mediators.

Increased circulation brings white blood cells and nourishment to the site of injury or infection so that invading pathogens are killed and damage may be repaired. Characteristic signs of inflammation include pain (dolor), heat (calor), swelling (tumor) and redness (rubor).

While some inflammation is beneficial and appropriate for healing, chronic or excessive inflammation, serving no purpose produces damage. Chronic inflammation has a bad reputation because it is implicated in various disease processes including but not limited to soft tissue swelling and chemical mediators involved in inflammation can also irritate nerve endings, contributing to pain.

It is a well-known fact that different foods are metabolized differently, some promoting inflammation and others reducing it. The purpose of the anti-inflammatory diet is to promote optimal health and healing by choosing foods that reduce inflammation.

If one can successfully control excessive inflammation through natural means (like through diet), it reduces one's dependence on anti-inflammatory medications that have unwanted and unhealthy side effects and don't solve the underlying problem.

While anti-inflammatory medications (such as NSAIDs) are a quick fix to ease symptoms, they ultimately weaken the immune system by damaging the gastrointestinal tract which plays an important role in immune system function

You have chosen to take your life and your health back and eat an anti-inflammatory diet. Many people are making the same choice to fight the effects of obesity, diabetes, arthritis and other inflammatory conditions. As is the case with any dietary change, after a time, the control once assumed over the foods eaten can grown lax.

Inflammation is a normal biological process with a purpose. However, excessive inflammation, serving no purpose can be damaging. In this GUIDE, you'll learn the basics of the anti- inflammatory diet to reduce inflammation naturally.

Chapter 1

What Is Inflammation?

Inflammation can be defined as the body's natural defense to infections and injuries. When something goes wrong the body's immune system goes to work to inflame the area, which serves to get rid of the invader or to heal the wound. Inflammation can cause pain, swelling, redness, and warmth, but this goes away as soon as the problem is solved. This is good inflammation.

Then we have chronic inflammation, the type that's familiar to people with rheumatoid arthritis (RA), lupus, psoriatic arthritis, and other types of "inflammatory" arthritis. Chronic inflammation is the type that will not go away.

All the types of arthritis that are mentioned above are a disorder of the immune system creates inflammation and then doesn't know when to shut off. Inflammatory arthritis, chronic inflammation can have serious consequences, permanent disability and tissue damage can be one if it isn't treated properly. Inflammation has been linked to a full host of other medical conditions.

Inflammation has been found to contribute to atherosclerosis, which is when fat builds up on the lining of arteries, raising the risk of heart attacks.

Also, high levels of inflammation proteins have been found in the blood of people with heart disease. Inflammation has also been linked to obesity, diabetes, asthma, depression, and even Alzheimer disease and cancer.

Scientists think that a constant level of inflammation in the body, even if the level is low, can have a number of negative effects.

Research shows that diet can reduce inflammation; in theory an inflammation-lowering diet should have an effect on a wide range of health conditions.

Researchers have looked for clues in the eating habits of our early ancestors to discover which foods might benefit us the most. They believe those habits are more in tune to our eating habits with how the body processes and uses what we eat and drink.

Our ancestor's diet consisted of wild lean meats (venison or boar) and wild plants (green leafy vegetables, fruits, nuts, and berries). There were no cereal grains until the agriculture revolution (about 10,000 years ago).

There was very little dairy, and there were no processed or refined foods. Our diets are usually are high in meat, saturated (or bad) fats, and processed foods, and there is very little exercise.

Nearly everything we eat is available close by or as far away as our computer and the click of a mouse.

Our diet and lifestyles are way out of whack with how our bodies are made from the inside out. While our genetic make-up has changed very little from our early beginnings, our diet and lifestyles have changed a great deal and the changes have gotten worse over the last 50 to 100 years.

Our genes haven't had a chance to adapt. We aren't giving our bodies the right kind of fuel, it's as though we think of our bodies as engines in a jet plane when instead they are like the engine in the very first planes. There are some foods that we are putting into our

bodies, especially because we are eating way too much of them, that are affecting our health in a bad way.

There are two nutrients in our diets that have attracted attention, are omega-3 fatty acids and omega-6 fatty acids have been part of our diets for thousands of years. They are components in just about all of our many cells and are important for normal growth and development.

Both of these acids play a role in inflammation. In several studies it was found that certain sources of omega 3's in particular, help to reduce the inflammation process and that omega 6's will raise it.

Now this is the problem, the average American eats on average about 15 times more omega 6's than omega 3's.

While our very early ancestor's ate omega 6's and omega 3's in equal ratio, and it is believed that this is what helped to balance their ability to turn inflammation on and off.

The imbalance of omega 3's and omega 6's in our diets is believed to contribute to the excess of inflammation in our bodies.

Vegetable oils such as corn oil, safflower oil, sunflower oil, cottonseed oil, soybean oil, and the products made from them, such as margarine, are loaded with omega 6's. Even many of the processed snack foods that are so readily available today are full of these oils.

Based on the best information of the time, was to use vegetable oils like those mentioned above instead of foods with saturated fats such as butter and lard. It looks like the conse q uences of that advice may have contributed to the increased consumption of omega 6's and therefore causing an imbalance of omega 3's and omega 6's.

You can find omega 6's in other common foods such as meats and egg yolks. The omega 6 found in meat is the fatty acids that come from grain-fed animals such as cows, lambs, pigs and chickens.

Most of the meat sold in America is grain fed unlike their grass-fed cousins who contain less of those fatty acids.

Wild game such as venison and boar are lower in omega 6's and fat and higher in omega 3's than the meat that comes from the supermarkets where we shop.

You can get omega 3s in both animal and plant food. Our bodies can convert omega 3s from animal sources into anti-inflammatory compounds more easily than the omega 3s from plant sources. Plant foods contain hundreds of other healthful compounds many of which that are anti-inflammatory, so don't discount them all together.

There are many foods that are high in omega 3s and that include fatty fish, especially fish from cold waters. Of course everyone knows about salmon but did you know that you can also find omega 3s in mackerel, anchovies, sardines, herring, striped bass, and bluefish.

It's also widely known that wild fish are better sources of omega 3s than the farm raised ones. You can also buy eggs that have been enriched with omega 3 oils. There are several excellent sources of omega 3s in plants that are leafy greens (like kale, Swiss chard, and spinach) as well as flaxseed, wheat germ, walnuts, and their oils.

You can also get omega 3s in supplements (often as fish oil); this source has been shown to be beneficial in some instances. You should take with your doctor before you take a fish oil supplement because it can interact with some medications and under certain circumstances can increase the risk of bleeding.

I take a prescribed omega 3 supplement because my doctor had told me that the ones you get in the supermarket or health food store are not pure, they have other additives that do absolutely nothing to help. There are other fats that are contributors to clogged arteries, the "bad" or saturated fats found in meats and high-fat dairy foods, these are called pro-inflammatory.

Transfats

There are also the Trans fats that are relatively new to the cause of heart disease. These Trans fats can be found in processed convenience and snack foods and can be spotted by reading the labels.

They can be identified as partially hydrogenated oils, often soybean oil or cottonseed oil. But, they can also occur naturally in small amounts in animal foods.

The thought is that they contribute to the pro-inflammatory activities in our bodies and the amounts we eat today are staggering.

Antioxidants are substances that prevent inflammation causing "free radicals" from over taking our bodies. Plant foods such as fruits, vegetables (including beans), nuts, and seeds carry high amounts of antioxidants.

Extra-virgin olive oil and walnut oil are very good sources of antioxidants, also.

These foods have long been considered the basics for good health, and can be found in fruits and vegetables with colorful and vibrant pigments. The more colorful the plant, the better they are for you, from green vegetables, especially leafy ones, to low-starch vegetables, such as broccoli and cauliflower, to berries, tomatoes, and brightly colored orange and yellow fruits and vegetables.

We don't have to revert back completely to the caveman to eat the anti-inflammatory way to benefit from the anti-inflammatory diet. Just eating a healthful diet that is recommended today is right on track.

Our chief strategy should be to balance the amount of modern day foods with the foods of long ago, which were rich in the inflammation reducing foods.

Really, all we have to do is replace foods rich in omega 6 with foods rich in omega 3, cutting down on how much meat and poultry we eat while eating oily fish a couple of times a week and adding more varieties of colorful fruits and vegetables, and while whole grains were not a part of our early ancestor's diet, it should be included in ours.

Be sure that it is whole grains and not refined grains because they contain many beneficial nutrients and inflammation-tempering compounds. Researchers have found that eating a lot of foods high in sugar and white flour may promote inflammation, although there is more studying that needs to be done on the subject.

Chapter 2

Inflammation and problems

Inflammation is a good thing. It is the natural way your body responds to threats such as infections or wounds. We have all seen inflammation at work when we have pain and redness at an injury. We say it looks inflamed, and it literally is, because injury activates the inflammatory response.

When inflammation lasts for long periods of time, we call it chronic, and it can cause problems. Some common causes of chronic inflammation include allergies, autoimmune disease, periodontal disease, arthritis and other diseases that activate the immune system over time. Even obesity is inflammatory, because fat cells give off chemicals called cytokines that trigger inflammation.

Chronic inflammation causes damage to the endothelial lining of arteries, which can lead to atherosclerosis and heart disease. There is also evidence that it contributes to type 2 diabetes, Alzheimer's disease and a growing number of other chronic diseases that are common in modern, western societies.

Chronic inflammation is a type of inflammation that silently attacks the body causing disease and degeneration, and is also known as "silent inflammation". As the connection between silent inflammation and a host of diseases becomes clearer, the case for dietary and lifestyle changes that can combat inflammation has become stronger.

While it was always known that some conditions such as arthritis and acne were a result of acute inflammation in the body, there is mounting evidence that silent inflammation plays a role in heart disease, Alzheimer's, diabetes and some cancers, as well as in the ageing process. Chronic inflammation can be present undetected in your body for years, until it manifests in disease.

Silent inflammation has been linked with the buildup of cholesterol deposits in the arteries which can lead to heart disease. In a similar way, the risk of Alzheimer's disease increases with inflammation of brain tissue, as this results in the buildup of amyloid plaque deposits in the brain.

Having type 2 diabetes, or eating sugary foods contributes to silent inflammation in the body as a result of elevated blood sugar and insulin levels. Recent studies have also confirmed the link between inflammation and several types of cancers.

Making the necessary lifestyle changes to fight inflammation, can protect you from it's devastating effects.

There are molecules in the body called prostaglandins which play an important role in inflammation. It has been found that of the three main types of prostaglandins, two of them (PG-E1 and PG-E3) have an anti-inflammatory effect, while the third type (PG-E2) actually promotes inflammation.

Inflammation triggers a response from the immune system. Initially inflammation is beneficial as it is used for protection but a lot of the time inflammation can lead to further inflammation (Chronic) which leads to big health problems.

What causes the inflammation in the first place?

- Chronic infections Obesity
- Environmental toxins (food, water & air)
- Physiological stress
- Intensive /endurance training Physical trauma
- Age
- Autoimmune disease

If you notice that in the brackets for environmental toxins is food.

What are the symptoms?

The symptoms of inflammation vary with what is causing it. You may even have no symptoms at all, as in the case of obesity. Here are some examples of specific disease related symptoms:

- Arthritis, rheumatoid arthritis (joint pain, stiffness, swelling)
- Crohn's disease or ulcerative colitis (abdominalpain and cramping, fever, diarrhea)
- Psoriasis or eczema (redness) Allergies (respiratory symptoms, hives)

More subtle, early indicators of problems could include headaches, muscles aches, fatigue, muscle stiffness, nausea, vomiting, diarrhea or constipation, gas, abdominal discomfort and even emotional problems including depression.

These could be related to food sensitivities and intolerances. The most common food intolerances include dairy (lactose), wheat (gluten), yeast, soy, corn, eggs and even some artificial sweeteners.

You can find out if you have inflammation by having your C- reactive protein levels tested. The high sensitivity C-reactive protein, is the preferred indicator of chronic, low-grade inflammation.

What should I do if I have high levels of C- reactive protein?

If your C-reactive protein levels are high, you will first want to talk to your doctor to find out if there is an underlying infection, allergy, autoimmune disorder or other contributing disease. If not, your excess weight could be the cause and weight loss is your best line of defense. If you are a smoker, that could also be contributing to the problem.

Some of our bodies are already on fire on the inside, and some of our habits are the same as throwing petrol on that fire. Inflammation is the body's biological response of attempting to protect itself. It aims to remove harmful stimuli, such as pathogens, damaged cells and irritants; this is the first step of the healing process.

When there is an imbalance in the body between these prostaglandins, inflammation can result.

Prostaglandins are made in the body from essential fatty acids.

You can assist your body in making anti-Inflammatory prostaglandins by eating vegetables, nuts, grains and seeds such as sesame and sunflower seeds. On the other hand, foods that cause a spike in insulin levels, such as sugary foods, or foods with a high Glycemic load promote production of PG-E2 and increase inflammation.

Chapter 3

How Do Foods Influence Inflammation?

Inflammation can also be influenced by the foods you eat. Research has shown that certain foods trigger inflammation and others suppress it.

Some of the foods that are pro-inflammatory include:

Animal fats (corn-fed beef, dark meat and skin of poultry, pork, duck

Hydrogenated fats (trans fat)

Fried foods (fried in saturated, hydrogenated or polyunsaturated fats)

Sweets (sugar, candy, cookies, cakes, ice cream, donuts, sweet drinks)

Refined grains (white bread, pasta, white rice)

Processed foods (chips, crackers, fries, cold cuts, hot dogs, canned meats)

Dairy products (especially full fat milk, cheese, sour cream, cream cheese, cream)

Some people may also need to avoid the nightshades (potatoes, tomatoes, eggplant, peppers)

Here are some of the best anti-inflammatory foods:

Fatty fish such as salmon, sardines, herring, trout and tuna (with omega 3 fatty acids)

Grass fed beef also contain some omega 3 fats (unlike corn-fed beef, mostly saturated fats)

Nuts and seeds (walnuts, flaxseed, almonds)

Monounsaturated fats (olive oil, canola oil, avocados), by replacing polyunsaturated fats

Turmeric (part of most curry dishes)

Ginger, used in Asian cuisine (also helps control nausea)

Whole grains (except wheat, barley and rye if you are gluten intolerant)

Foods that have high antioxidant levels also tend to reduce inflammation, possibly by reducing the damage that stimulates inflammation. Antioxidants are prolific in brightly and darkly colored fruits and vegetables.

Some of the best sources of antioxidants include:

- Berries: nblueberries, raspberries, blackberries, cranberries, strawberries, cherries,
- Beans: Red beans, kidney beans, pinto and black beans

- Herbs: oregano, basil, sage, marjoram, thyme, dill, garlic, dry mustard
- Spices: cinnamon, cloves, cumin, turmeric, ginger

- Nuts: pecans, walnuts, pistachios
- Green tea is rich in both antioxidants and anti-inflammatory compounds
- Coffee, cocoa (or dark chocolate) and red wine (but caffeine and alcohol are inflammatory)
- Exotic fruits: acai, gogi, pomegranate, papaya, pineapple

Eating more of these anti-inflammatory and high antioxidant foods can help calm chronic inflammation and by doing so, reduce your risk for chronic diseases. Find ways to make these foods a part of your everyday diet and you will not only be protecting your body from disease, but you may find that some of your aches and pains improve.

A typical anti-inflammatory diet focuses on fighting inflammation through the consumption of foods that lower insulin levels.

To actively reduce inflammation, you should therefore eat foods that have a low Glycemic load, such as whole grains, vegetables and lentils, and consume healthy fats such as nuts, seeds, fish, extra virgin olive oil and fish. Spices such as turmeric, ginger, and hot peppers also reduce inflammation.

At the same time, you also need to reduce consumption of foods that are pro-inflammatory, such as red meat, egg yolks and shellfish. Sugar is a key culprit in inflammation, and therefore you should also cut back on sugary foods. Inflammation can also be reduced by taking supplements such as fish oils which are high in Omega 3 fatty acids.

Chapter 4

What Is An Anti-Inflammatory Diet?

In general, an anti-inflammatory diet consists of fresh, whole foods which do not contain triggers for inflammation and are loaded with molecules that actually neutralize inflammation in your body.

The amounts of knowledge we have on how the body works and how our ancestor's ate is helping to confirm the old adage: "You are what you eat." But, there is still more we need to learn before we can prescribe any one anti-inflammatory diet.

Our genetic makeup and the severity of our health condition will determine the benefits we get from an anti-inflammatory diet and unfortunately there is doubt that there will be one diet that fits us all.

Also, what we eat or don't eat is just a small part of the whole story. We are not as physically active as our ancestors and physical activity has its own anti-inflammatory effects. Our ancestors were also much leaner than we are and body fat is active tissue that can make inflammatory producing compounds.

Anti-inflammatory eating is a way of selecting foods that are more in tune with what the body actually needs. We can achieve a more balanced diet by going back to our roots.

If you look at the diet of the people of the Bible, you will find that they, like our caveman ancestors, were more active and their diets consisted of much the same things as our caveman ancestors.

They also had no choice but to walk everywhere they wanted to go, there was no such thing as cars or trucks. While we have it easier today, our health has suffered greatly from it.

According to some proponents of an Anti-Inflammatory diet, low grade inflammation may be at the root of everything from heart disease and diabetes to arthritis and Alzheimer's disease. Inflammation is the way the body's immune system responds to attack, injury or infection. Symptoms include swelling, pain, sometimes loss of movement or function and red coloration.

The immune system is a complex system of organs, tissues and specialized cells that protects the body from invasions by viruses, bacteria and allergens as well as harmful insiders such as infected cells and toxins.

Autoimmune diseases are a result of the system turning on itself and damaging tissue and creating substances that result in chronic health conditions. Type 1 diabetes, arthritis, cancer, multiple sclerosis and systemic lupus are all examples of autoimmune diseases.

The immune system response to an unhealthy diet can lead to this chronic inflammation. Although an anti-inflammatory diet cannot eradicate inflammation, it purportedly can reduce the inflammation that causes autoimmune disease.

Aren't there drugs that can do this?

Yes, of course there are. That is what NSAIDs (Non-Steroidal Anti- Inflammatory Drugs) are for. And they work; sort of. There are mixed reports on NSAIDs effect on inflammation.

Some evidence shows that people on NSAIDs for long periods have a lower incidence of autoimmune disease. Other studies show that long term use can actually lead to cardiovascular problems.

Any food with refined sugar or white flour in it tends to be inflammatory. Fast foods, deep fried foods, fat and processed foods all are considered inflammatory.

An anti-inflammatory diet would exclude these items and include fresh fruits and vegetables, Omega 3 oils such as found in salmon, and a minimum of red meat. In other words this diet is no different from what we have constantly been told is a healthy diet. There are popular diets that are good examples.

Most people who experience inflammation have heard all about the medications that are available to cure the pain and swelling that can occur during a flare up.

But how many know that there are some great anti-inflammatory foods that can affect how you feel and reduce the pain associated with inflammation. Following an anti-inflammatory diet will help you beat inflammation naturally.

Inflammation is a swelling that may cause pain, discoloration and even the loss of movement. Usually most people experience severe inflammation when they are the sufferers of arthritis and when they have problems like heart disease and strokes.

Usually your doctor will recommend that you get sleep and exercise in moderation. He may also suggest lowering your weight and taking steroid based drugs or undergoing joint replacement surgery.

The medications do work fairly well in reducing the inflammation but often come with some serious side effects, such as ulcers and kidney problems. This may make you wonder if they are worth taking and whether using them is trading one illness for another.

Just like there are some foods that decrease inflammation, there are some that will increase the likelihood that you will get inflammation.

These foods are junk foods, fast foods, sugar, and fatty meats. Processed foods that contain Trans and saturated fats also increase the risk of inflammation.

Other large contributors of saturated fats are dairy products and eggs. By simply choosing low fat milk, low fat cheese and leaner cuts of meat, you can lower the risks of inflammation, as well as cut down on the chances of chronic disease and obesity. Other foods that increase inflammation include presweetened cereals and soft drinks.

In addition to these, there are foods that are high in sugar and foods that come from the plants labeled as nightshade type. These add to the risk of discomfort associated with inflammation.

Eating whole fruits and vegetables will give you the natural healing factors. However, not all vegetables work that way. Potatoes, eggplant and tomatoes can actually make inflammation worse.

So remember the best foods to have are whole fruits, fresh vegetables, lean meats, low fat milk and cheese, as well as fruit and vegetable juices that contain carrots and celery. These types of foods will reduce inflammation and help you get on with your life without pain. Eating right will help you beat inflammation naturally.

Chapter 5

The Benefits of An Anti-Inflammatory Diet

People suffering from obesity have inflammation issues. Diabetes, arthritis and asthma are all associated with inflammation in the body. Not to mention the link to certain heart conditions and cancers.

Reducing the inflammation in your body with an anti-inflammation diet can cause an immediate change to how you feel, not to mention the long term effects of the dietary change on health and well-being.

The first step to adopting an anti-inflammatory diet is to understand the effects of foods on the body. Food provides nutrients and vitamins the body needs to survive.

The idea of eating to live not living to eat is a huge push for the weight loss community, but this idea should not just be followed when needing to lose a few pounds.

Certain foods have high concentrations of anti-oxidants and natural anti-inflammatory nutrients that may reduce the effect of inflammation on the body. It is these foods that cornerstone the anti- inflammatory diet.

The Role of Omega 3 and Other Fatty Acids

Fatty acids are present in many foods that contain oil. The best natural source is fish like salmon and sardines. However, Omega 6 fatty acids are prevalent in western diets over Omega 3s. This is

because common eaten foods like chicken, turkey, eggs, nuts and vegetable oils are rich in Omega 6 fatty acids.

What people don't realize, however, is that these fatty acids need to be balanced with Omega 3s for optimal health and anti-inflammatory action. Most western diets include 10 times more Omega 6s than Omega 3s. Some diets include as much as 30 times more. The optimal ratio is 4 parts Omega 6 to every 1 part Omega 3.

Increasing Omega 3 fatty acids in the diet can reduce inflammation in the body and thus reduce the effect of this condition on health and general well-being. Foods rich in Omega 3s include fish oil, kiwi, black raspberry and various nuts.

The most readily available source of Omega 3s is flaxseeds. Many people mistake fish oils for the best source, but flaxseed oils tend to have the most readily available Omega 3s that make absorption in the body easier.

Flaxseed oils contain about 55% ALA (alpha-linoleic acid) which is an Omega 3 fatty acid.

Fatty Meats Be Gone

Another simple change to reduce inflammation in the body is the reduction of fatty meats. Red meat is the worst of all meats for people suffering from inflammation. Choosing a leaner cut or a leaner alternative is a good option. Bison and venison are two options that tend to contain less fat.

Grass fed cows also have fewer inflammatory characteristics on the body. Fish, lean chicken, turkey, soybeans, tofu and soy milk are all lean choices for decreasing inflammation.

But some of these meats tend to be higher in Omega 6s. To combat the fatty acid imbalance that may be increasing inflammation, try cooking these meats in olive oil or adding flaxseed oil to the final dish to boost Omega 3s.

The Danger of Processed Foods

The worst food to eat when suffering from inflammation is a processed carbohydrate. These foods offer very little nutritional value and should be replaced with whole grain alternatives. All flour is wheat based, but processed flour is stripped of the healthy grain wholeness and bleached.

What are left are empty calories sure to swell the body even more. Simply replacing white bread with whole grain bread and white flour with whole wheat flour that is unbleached can make a big difference in how your body reacts to your diet.

Chapter 6

The Biggest Struggles Of An Anti-Inflammatory Diet

Everyone wants to feel better and live in better health. One of the easiest ways to achieve that is by switching from a traditional western diet to an anti-inflammatory diet. Making the change is easy, but much like a diet plan, sticking with the food changes and watching what you eat can be difficult.

Fast Food and Your Inflammation

Fast food is a huge hindrance to the anti-inflammatory diet. Foods that are high in fat tend to increase inflammatory substances in the body for three to four hours after the meal.

If the same number of calories eaten in one fast food sitting were eaten as fresh fruits, vegetables and lean meats, this effect would not occur. Free radicals, cell killers that compound inflammation problems, can also be increased by 175% after eating fast food.

The Alternative –

The best alternative to fast food is a replacement, anti-inflammatory diet. Take the Big Mac from McDonald's into consideration. This sandwich can be made from lean ground turkey and a whole grain bun.

The "special" sauce can be mixed up with lower carbohydrate ketchup, olive oil mayonnaise and sugar free relish. The result is a tasty alternative with a significantly lower fat count.

Red Meat, Milk and Your Inflammation

Science has long fought to connect red meat with certain forms of cancer. Little did they know the research would lead to a link between this common dinner protein and inflammation. Researchers believe the body reacts to certain chemical aspects of red meat and milk in a protective manner.

If the body believes these are foreign substances, the immune system will kick in and inflammation occurs. Imagine eating red meat once a day and drinking two or three glasses of milk. The body would live in a state of constant or chronic inflammation which could cause health problems over time.

The Alternative

Lean poultry, beef and fish are all part of a healthy diet. Beef is a great source of iron, so eliminating it is not a necessity. But, choosing the leanest of cuts is essential to good health. The best meats are lean proteins and beans.

Trans Fats and Your Inflammation

A hidden source of body inflammation is the trans fatty acid. While many people know a bit about this type of fat, few understand the effects on the body. Fast food, baked goods, prepackaged meals and margarine are often good sources of trans fat.

After entering the body, these fats can increase the risk of coronary artery disease, insulin resistance, diabetes and heart failure. Increased risk of stroke due to abnormally high lipid levels is also common. While many foods will claim to be trans-fat free, that is not the entire truth.

According to labeling guidelines, these foods can contain up to 0.5 grams of trans fats per serving and still mark the product as "trans fat free". These small amounts will add up over time if the diet is rich in processed foods, margarine and baked goods.

The Alternative –

Natural fats like whole butter and olive oil have no trans fats. Choosing these in place of hydrogenated oils and margarine is a good first step. When it comes to foods cooked in trans-fat, there is no choice but to eliminate these from the diet all together.

Many people choose to adopt an anti-inflammatory diet by baking their own snacks and cooking "fast food" style meals at home.

Chapter 7

Who Needs An Anti-Inflammatory Diet?

Inflammation is often associated with injury. You stub your toe and the toe swells. This is the basic inflammatory reaction. Some people even understand that redness around a cut is also a form of inflammation that the immune system uses to heal the injury.

What is not commonly known is the fact that inflammation occurs inside the body as well. When the body exists in an inflammatory state, risk of illness, cancer and heart conditions can increase. An anti-inflammatory diet is an easy way to combat this aftereffect and reduce risk today.

This is the most common statement and the least correct. Inflammation affects every person in the world at some point in their life. In western cultures, like the United States, a huge portion of the population is affected by inflammation every day.

Being overweight or obese is the most common inflammatory condition. It is this inflammatory response that could be the cause of some weight related conditions like diabetes.

When fat cells grow, they take up the free space around the organs. Blood flow can be constricted and the body often feels as though it needs to fight to function normally. When the body feels threatened, inflammation occurs as a natural, healing response.

Unfortunately, unlike the small cut that will heal in a few, short days. Obesity takes time to correct and the longer the body lives inflamed, the greater the risk of long term effects.

In the case of obesity, changing the diet by reducing calories will reduce body weight and thus reduce the inflammation in the body. This is the simplest benefit of an anti-inflammatory diet. However, people who are obese or overweight are not the only people who can benefit from an anti-inflammatory diet.

There are many illnesses and conditions caused by inflammation. These include asthma, arthritis, inflammatory bowel syndrome, pelvic inflammatory disease, endometriosis, diabetes, COPD, Psoriasis, Colitis, and Lupus - just to name a few. All-in-all, there are nearly 40 autoimmune conditions currently accepted by the medical community that are affected by inflammation.

The first step is to make dietary changes to reduce food based inflammation.

Processed foods, fast foods and prepackaged foods can cause increased inflammation in the body.

Replacing these foods with lean meats, whole grains and healthy fats will make a tremendous different in how the body reacts to inflammation. In addition, if weight is a problem, reducing weight while changing to an anti-inflammatory diet can increase the benefits exponentially.

Changing to an anti-inflammatory diet does not have to be in reaction to a disease or illness. Prevention is the best choice and the anti-inflammatory diet can reduce the risk of contracting many of the listed illnesses.

When the body feels as though it needs to fight for survival, inflammation occurs, so offering healthy foods that have an inflammatory effect is a great choice for all people including those who are young, healthy and feel they do not need an anti- inflammatory diet.

Most chronic diseases are a result of a lifestyle of affluence that affords us the luxury of being able to eat the wrong foods in the wrong amounts at the wrong times. These food choices set in play a host of processes in your body that produce inflammation from a multitude of sources.

In addition, many of us are genetically programmed to produce excessive inflammation when exposed to common irritant sources such as smoke, chemicals and poor dietary choices.

Some of us produce so much inflammation that we have autoimmune disorders such as lupus, multiple sclerosis, rheumatoid arthritis, psoriasis and colitis.

How exactly do poor food choices produce inflammation?

Packaged and highly processed foods as well as fast foods are some of the worst culprits. They are also some of the food choices most widely available. Designed for convenience, these foods are loaded with trans-fat to extend their shelf life as well as change their taste and texture.

A trans-fat is created from a natural, saturated fat - another less than healthy fat.

That saturated fat is "transformed" into a trans-fat via a process called trans-hydrogenation. This transformed fat is chemically different enough from a natural fat that, when incorporated into your

body tissues, it creates a cascade of chemicals called cytokines. Cytokines are molecules responsible for producing inflammation throughout your body.

Foods that are loaded with refined sugars are also inflammatory.

Cakes, cookies and doughnuts are examples of foods that are rapidly digested by your body, releasing large amounts of glucose. This glucose is rapidly absorbed by your body, causing a high blood glucose level. Your body in turn releases a surge of insulin to help normalize your blood glucose levels.

This surge of insulin combined with high blood glucose levels causes your body to release cytokines, inflammatory molecules, as well. Each surge of glucose actually signals your body to store fat. Guess what? Fat tissue becomes physiologically active and begins to release these same inflammatory molecules, cytokines, as well.

Refined grains - grains stripped of fiber and vital nutrients- also create inflammation. A whole grain is a molecule composed of large amounts of glucose linked together and encapsulated with a fiber coating. This fiber coating makes the digestion and release of glucose a slow and steady process.

When the outer fiber coating is stripped away to create a smooth and creamy texture, glucose molecules are readily available for rapid digestion and absorption into your body. This rapid surge of glucose into your system again is the trigger for the inflammatory cascade.

Certain grains have the ability to produce inflammation in certain individuals. Wheat, oats, barley and rye are all grains that contain significant amounts of a protein substance called gluten.

Gluten makes foods, like bread, crunchy on the outside and soft on the inside.

Yet this same gluten is very inflammatory in individuals genetically challenged in digesting gluten. Symptoms can be as severe as pain, bloating, diarrhea and malnutrition or as mild as nausea or lack of energy. Eliminating these specific grains from your diet is often the key to controlling this type of inflammation.

Phytonutrients are found in most fruits and vegetables, responsible for their colorful appearance. These huge molecules have antioxidant as well as anti-inflammatory properties.

This means they neutralize the oxidative stress that your body generates daily, leading to inflammation. Healthy fats found in cold- water, fatty fish, flax seed and nuts can also diminish the amount of inflammation produced by your body as well.

Cooking oils such as olive oil and canola oil also help your body fight and neutralize inflammation. Certain vitamins and minerals - vitamin A,D, E and C as well as zinc, selenium and copper - are found in abundance in fresh, whole foods. These antioxidants also neutralize oxidative stress and dampen the formation of inflammation.

Eliminating fast foods as well as packaged foods is the first step of the anti-inflammatory diet.

Eliminating foods with refined sugars and processed grains is the second step.

Eating generous amounts daily of fresh fruit and vegetables and moderate amounts of whole grains and lean protein as well as healthy fats found in fish, seeds and nuts is the foundation of the anti-inflammatory diet. Then for select individuals, reducing or eliminating grains, especially gluten-containing grains, is the final step.

So just who should eat an anti-inflammatory diet?

Obviously, anyone who suffers from an inflammatory condition such as autoimmune disorders (lupus, multiple sclerosis, rheumatoid arthritis, colitis.) or allergic disorders (asthma, eczema) will benefit from the anti-inflammatory diet.

Most people with chronic pain (headaches, back pain, neck pain, knee pain, joint pains, nerve pains, muscle pains) have elements of inflammation involved in their pain and will benefit too.

Irritable bowel syndrome and common digestive disorders such as acid reflux improve with the anti-inflammatory diet. Yet surprisingly, anyone suffering with chronic degenerative disorders (arthritis, diabetes, heart disease, obesity and even cancer) will benefit as well from this diet.

Finally, anyone interested in preventing these degenerative diseases and achieving optimal health will benefit. In fact, the science confirms that eating to prevent inflammation not only prevents disease and maintains health but also keeps us looking and feeling younger. From children to the elderly, everyone can benefit from this powerful approach to eating.

Chapter 8

Anti-Inflammatory Foods to Add to Your Diet

High levels of inflammation can cause a number of health complications such as arthritis, joint pain, damage to blood vessels among others.

To combat this, it is important you eat foods that are anti- inflammatory. Such foods are readily available to add to your diet to curb inflammation. Here are some of the foods and suggestions to help and keep harmful inflammation at bay:

Whole Grains

When it comes to whole grains it is better you consume your grains as whole grains and not refined or pasta. Research has shown that whole grains contain a high amount of fibre which reduces the inflammatory marker in blood known as C-reactive protein.

Dark Leafy Greens

Dark leafy vegetables such as spinach and kale have high concentrations of vitamin E and minerals such as calcium and iron. Studies show that vitamin E helps in protecting your body from inflammatory molecules known as cytokines. Additionally, dark leafy greens have a high amount of disease fighting phytochemicals.

Fatty Fish

Oily fish such as salmon and tuna are foods that are anti-inflammatory as they contain high amounts of omega 3 fatty acids. The fatty acids are known to help joint inflammation, so make sure you get plenty of omega 3. Another important fact about omega 3 is you must get it in your food because the body cannot make it within its system.

Soy

Soybeans contain isoflavones compounds which help the negative effects of inflammation on joints. However, it is good you avoid heavily processed soy products as they may contain additives and preservatives. Instead, include soy milk and soy beans into your regular diet.

Nuts

Nuts such as almonds and walnuts are rich in vitamin E, calcium and fibre. All nuts are full of antioxidants which can help the body in repairing the damages caused by inflammation.

Berries

Berries are low in fat and calories but rich in antioxidants. Their anti- inflammatory anthocyanins compound in them has many good qualities. This helps to prevent you from developing arthritis.

Green Tea

Green tea as well has anti-inflammatory flavonoids; this reduces the onset of inflammation and minimizes the risk of certain cancers. It shouldn't be underestimated for many other health benefits. It can reactivate skin cells making skin appear brighter. Drink it regularly and use some honey as a sweetener instead of sugar.

Low Fat Dairy

Low fat dairy such as yogurt contains probiotics which can prevent inflammation. Additionally, dairy foods that are anti-inflammatory such as skim milk with high calcium and vitamin D are important for everyone since apart from having anti-inflammatory properties, they strengthen your bones also.

Ginger and Garlic

Ginger and garlic are foods that are anti-inflammatory. Both are known to lower body inflammation, control blood sugar levels and help your body in fighting certain infections. Selenium and sulphur in garlic is an essential compound for a healthy immune system. It is also one of the top anti-aging foods you can eat.

Turmeric and Sweet Potato

Turmeric has natural anti-inflammatory compounds called curcumin which is known to turn off NF-kappa B protein that triggers the process of inflammation.

On the other hand, sweet potato is a good source of fibre, vitamin B 6, vitamin C, complex carbohydrates and better carotene.

These ingredients help to heal inflammation in your body. These are some of many foods that are anti-inflammatory which can help you in reducing joint pain and arthritis caused by inflammation. Add them to your diet.

In addition, also eat steam leafy green vegetables so none of the nutrients are lost. Stay away from salt and cheese. You can make delicious shakes by combining fruits and vegetables.

For example: carrots and apples are a healthy combination, and include anti-oxidants which are an important element in your diet regimen. Ensure when eating any of the meats specified, you remove the skin as well as trimming the fat.

When eating nuts, choose almonds, walnuts, pecans, pine nuts, or hazelnuts. Roasting them, before consumption, releases essential oils which are most beneficial.

Herbs, except salt, have medicinal properties. Some of the more popular spices such as turmeric, ginger, cinnamon and oregano are often recommended by physicians.

Beans, peas and legumes, such as lentils, kidney beans, and chickpeas, to name a few, are very high in protein and are consider high fiber foods. Tip: Beans and escarole is not only a delicious and satisfying dinner, but extremely healthy as well.

Green tea is an antioxidant; two cups a day will suffice. Another anti- oxidant is extra virgin olive oil, and includes omega 9 fatty acids. Tip: This oil can also be used on your skin to achieve suppleness.

All of these anti-inflammatory foods have been touted by experts as being the most comprehensive and effective diet available. While there are other diet plans which offer similar results, depending upon your own personal circumstances, any diet rich in protein, oils and fiber is beneficial.

Using any of the aforementioned foods in your diet regimen can yield results, but it takes commitment and a willingness to persevere in order to achieve your goal to lose weight in a healthy and safe manner.

Spices

Turmeric would be on top of the list in reducing inflammation and joint pain. As well turmeric has a compound curcumin which is known for many health benefits and has the power to cure joint pain. It is best used in its natural powdery form and added to your diet when possible, the more the better.

Other important spices used for reducing inflammation are cinnamon, rosemary, garlic, ginger and oregano. These are high in polyphenols and bioflavonoids which help to reduce inflammation as well as fight off free radicals. Cayenne pepper is also known for its anti-inflammatory property and its capsicum content which is added to some creams for pain relief.

Grain

Whole grains which contain carbohydrates can also help in preventing spikes in the sugar level of the blood, as it is known that sugar promotes inflammation. However, use only non-refined whole grains, once processing has taken place all the goodness is lost, such as vitamins, minerals and fibre.

Among the best grains are oats: Whole oats, whole wheat, q uinoa, couscous and Bulgar. To take a multi supplement is of benefit, it can fill the spot of some foods you otherwise may not get from your diet as needed daily. However, your first priority must always be the diet, only than when taking a supplement you will get best value.

The right type of food and supplementation is crucial to treat arthritis, inflammation and joint pain. Multi vitamins that contain vitamin C, E, zinc, B 6, copper and boron are good to have included in your diet. It has been found that some nutrients deficiency in patients could

Be the cause of suffering from arthritis. There is also strong evidence that exercise is just as important as your diet.

Anyone suffering with arthritis pain, the last thing you would think about is exercise. You avoid moving as little as possible because every time you move it creates pain.

In fact, exercise is the alternative to joint pain relief, because it breaks the tendency to favor your joints and to avoid movement. Avoidance of movement and exercise will ultimately make the pain worse and weakens the body.

Chapter 9 Food To Avoid At All Costs On An Anti-Inflammation Diet

You have chosen to take your life and your health back and eat an anti-inflammatory diet. Many people are making the same choice to fight the effects of obesity, diabetes, arthritis and other inflammatory conditions. As is the case with any dietary change, after a time, the control once assumed over the foods eaten can grown lax.

Often, the same foods will creep back into the diet and reduce the efficacy of the anti-inflammatory diet. These are packaged foods, oil blends and margarine. Reducing protein and water intake are the remaining common factors.

Packaged foods are just plain bad for the body. Often these foods contain enough sodium and dietary fat for an entire day. While it may seem harmless to pop a meal in the microwave two or three times a week, the impact can be dramatic.

On average, prepackaged meals have between 700 and 1000 calories each. Just three meals a week can contribute an additional 3000 calories to the diet, not to mention the increases in fat and sodium. High fat meals cause inflammation in the body for hours after consumption and can lead to weight gain which is causes more inflammation.

Oil blends are easier on the budget than pure olive oil. These blends, however, can include oils that contain trans fats. These fats are unhealthy and should not be consumed at ALL in the diet. Saving a bit of money on the front side may be counteracting your good anti-inflammatory diet choices on the back side.

Margarine is cheaper and contains fewer calories than butter. Some people even believe that eating pure butter can cause an increase in cholesterol levels which may lead to stroke. This is NOT the case.

People who choose to eat very low carbohydrate diets, which often include high butter intakes, measure lower cholesterol numbers than their margarine or low fat eating peers.

Protein is expensive and lean protein can break the budget. When money is tight, buying that fatty burger to replace the 93/7 lean beef that was part of your anti-inflammatory diet may seem like a harmless choice. Fatty red meat is linked to an increased risk of cancer and causes inflammation in the body.

Instead, try replacing the burger, all together, will beans.

Water is the fluid of life and drinking water is the best choice for bettering overall health and decreasing inflammation.

Many people start off an anti-inflammatory diet by drinking a half gallon of water a day or more.

Over time, lax behavior may lead to increased caffeine intake and reduced water intake. Caffeine is linked to inflammation and can cause the anti-inflammatory diet to work less effectively at reducing inflammation.

The anti-inflammatory diet is not about strictly forbidding all foods that may increase inflammation. Deprivation is the number one reason people scrap new diets and return to old eating habits.

Instead of depriving, try healthier alternatives or simply reduce the number of times prepackaged foods, fatty red meats and trans fat based oils are eaten. Once in a while is not the problem. It is when that once in a while becomes every week or every day that inflammation may return even though you feel you are following an anti-inflammatory diet.

For some people, vegetables in the nightshade family may pose a concern.

 Examples of nightshade vegetables include tomatoes, peppers, potatoes and eggplant.

Nightshades contain alkaloids which are thought to exacerbate inflammation and joint damage in certain susceptible individuals with arthritis (though research is conflicting).

Thus, for some individuals, limiting or avoiding nightshade vegetables may be beneficial.

Fats:

Eat and Enjoy:

Enjoy healthy, anti-inflammatory fats including olive oil, coconut oil, avocados, nuts, salmon and sardines. In humans, there are two essential fatty acids, alpha-linolenic acid (an omega-3) and linoleic acid (an omega-6).

These are "essential" because they are re q uired for good health but the body does not synthesize them. Omega-3 fats are anti-inflammatory.

Omega-6 fats can be pro-inflammatory or anti-inflammatory (as it can be metabolized by two different pathways). Researchers suggest that keeping the ratio of omega-6 to omega-3 between 2:1 and 4:1 is best for health.

The modern diet tends to be high in omega-6 as it is abundantly available in cooking oils. Thus, including rich sources of omega-3 is important (such as fish, flax and walnuts especially).

Avoid / Limit:

Fats to limit or avoid include margarine, butter, shortening, hydrogenated oils, trans fats, saturated fats, and milk fat. Omega-6 fats are very high in corn oil, safflower oil and sunflower oil. Trans fats are linked with inflammatory disease.

Meat:

Eat and Enjoy:

In general, limit animal proteins because they tend to acidify the body and also promote inflammation. When selecting animal protein, enjoy fish, poultry (especially free-range and organically raised), lamb and omega-3 eggs.

Avoid / Limit:

Limit beef, pork, shellfish and factory farmed eggs. In general, grass- fed is superior to grain-fed. Avoid charred foods, smoked foods and cold cuts. Cold cuts contain nitrates and nitrites which promote cancer. Barbequed foods contain polycyclic aromatic hydrocarbons (PAHs) and heterocyclic amines (HCAs) which also promote cancer.

Dairy:

Eat and Enjoy:

Enjoy dairy substitutes in moderation (such as almond milk).

Avoid / Limit:

Avoid or limit dairy products in general. This includes milk, yogurt, cheese and ice cream. As we age, we lose the enzyme that digests dairy, resulting in lactose intolerance and inflammation. The milk protein, casein, is also acidifying which (despite what many people are brought up thinking) robs the bones of calcium.

Grains:

Eat and Enjoy:

Enjoy whole grains as opposed to refined grains. Refined grains are grains in which the germ and bran have been removed. This means there is loss of fiber, minerals and vitamins. In other words, the good stuff is removed in exchange for a longer shelf life. Some good examples of healthy grains include (organic) whole wheat/oats/bulgar/coucous, q uinoa and whole oats (like steel-cut oats).

Whole grains are also a rich source of complex carbohydrates. Complex carbohydrates (as opposed to simple sugars) will prevent spikes in your blood sugar level. Sugar promotes inflammation.

Avoid / Limit:

Avoid or limit refined carbohydrates such as white bread, pastries, sweet things and pastas.

Nuts:

Eat and Enjoy:

Enjoy nuts and nut butters such as almonds, walnuts, sesame seeds, pumpkin seeds and flax.

Avoid / Limit:

Avoid any specific nut allergies. Beverages:

Eat and Enjoy:

Enjoy plenty of pure, filtered water (avoiding chlorine, fluoride and other contaminants which are irritants that promote inflammation). Other great choices are lemon water and herbal teas.

Avoid / Limit:

Avoid sugary sodas, fruit juice (with sugar added) and milk. Spices:

Eat and Enjoy:

Many spices reduce inflammation. Some great examples are turmeric, oregano, rosemary, ginger, garlic and cinnamon. Bioflavenoids and polyphenols reduce inflammation and fight free radicals. Cayenne pepper is also anti-inflammatory, as it contains capsicum. Capsicum is often used in pain-relief creams.

Sweeteners:

Eat and Enjoy:

Enjoy stevia, molasses, maple syrup or honey as better alternatives for refined sugar.

Avoid / Limit

Avoid refined sugar, fructose and especially high fructose corn syrup which promote inflammation. Avoid artificial sweeteners.

Other:

Eat and Enjoy:

Enjoy fermented foods such as kimchi, miso soup and sauerkraut. Fermented foods are probiotic and help to rebuild the immune system by supporting healthy microflora in the gut and to reduce inflammation. Fermented foods also tend to be easy to digest and are also factories for B vitamins.

Avoid / Limit:

In general, eliminate processed foods, artificial colors, artificial flavors and preservatives. Also avoid foods that you have a known sensitivity or allergy to as this promotes inflammation.

Low grade sensitivities are easy to miss, so if you're unsure, have a food allergy test.

Some of the most common problem foods include wheat (gluten), corn, soy, milk and nuts.

Chapter 10 Anti-Inflammatory Herbs and Natural Sources

The concept of anti-inflammatory herbs is s very interesting one in the world of naturopathy and natural health. The reason why I gravitate towards them is because in the realm of inflammation and anti-inflammatory diets, they're a nice middle ground. Some people call for a total anti-inflammatory diet, eating only foods that promote the quelling of inflammation in the body.

Others are on the Standard American Diet, eating a host of foods that are known to cause inflammation in the body and aggravate many disorders and conditions. Anti-inflammatory herbs are a nice in-between. Foods in general are said to be either pro inflammatory or anti-inflammatory.

As you might have guessed, foods that are pro inflammatory will increase the amount of inflammation occurring in different parts of your body, will increase the pain associated with it, and may also increase your risk of having chronic disease. Foods pro inflammatory are most junk foods, sugars, fast foods, highly processed foods, and meats high in fat.

But that seems a bit excessive. That's why I love the idea of anti- inflammatory herbs.

They're a nice middle ground in the world of inflammation, allowing you to stay healthy in that arena without putting too much of a focus on inflammation in general.

Regularly eating some form of natural anti-inflammatory foods is key because it helps reduce the risk of things like arthritis and chronic autoimmune diseases. And due to the fact that herbal concoctions are generally fairly strong, anti-inflammatory herbs are a great addition to meals, as well as in supplements.

Herbs generally have a wide variety of health benefits, and because inflammation is a somewhat complex process in the body, herbs can affect inflammation in different ways. Inflammation, when carried beyond reasonable limits, can become a type of autoimmune condition.

It begins as negative stimuli causes white blood cells to activate in order to protect the area being negatively affected. Inflammation is necessary to the healing process, but chronic inflammation can cause lots of long term problems and is often excessive, like an allergic reaction.

Here are some of the best, most powerful anti-inflammatory herbs:

1.   Turmeric. Turmeric is a spice very common to most Indian foods. Though it has many other medicinal benefits, turmeric is a powerful anti-inflammatory herbs. But it takes a bit of time to start working, so if you don't like the taste of turmeric, you might want to think about taking it in capsule form.

2.   Ginger. Ginger is also a spice that is used very often in Asian cooking. This spice also has a potent flavor and takes a bit of time in order to take effect within the body.

Ginger is very versatile, being used in a range of both foods and drinks, so filling your diet with it shouldn't be too much of a challenge. You can drink ginger tea, ginger ale, use ginger in baked goods and spice meats with it.

3.   Omega 3 Essential Fatty Acids. Though these aren't technically herbs, omega 3 essential fatty acids are something that everyone needs more of in their diets. They're not only anti-inflammatory, they have a range of other medicinal benefits all across the body.

4.   Licorice. Licorice is another herb that is very effective in the world of anti-inflammation. This too is a great herb to take because of its diversity. Licorice is nice because it can be added to just about anything, like

candy, tea, baked goods, vegetables, meats, and more, making it easy to get a high daily dose.

5.   Mangosteen Juice. Mangosteen is a fruit native to Asia that has very powerful anti-inflammatory properties. Mangosteen juice is becoming more and more popular with persons who are suffering from the pain of arthritis, and mangosteen even has a very nice flavor. Many people substitute it for orange juice in their morning breakfast.

A few others worthy of note are:

- Pineapple juice

- Chamomile

- Black Seed Oil

- White Willow

- Red and Black Pepper

- St John's Wort

- Cilantro

- Cinnamon

- Garlic

- Cloves

Chapter 11 The Natural Anti-Inflammatory Diet Breakfast

One of the secrets of relieving pain and chronic inflammation understands the potential of your kitchen. This is the food your prepare in your home and eat to rebuild your body. Just open your fridge, pause, and look at what your body will be made of tomorrow.

In this chapter, I will create a wonderful natural anti-inflammatory and antioxidant breakfast that will give you energy and a great start to your day. Interested? Excellent.

First I would like to introduce you to what I consider to be the greatest culinary invention of the last hundred years. The magical blender. No, not the juicer which separates the vital fiber from everything. Nor the food processor which does no more than a good knife and spoon and takes away the meditation from cooking.

Several mornings each week start with the Hamilton Shake, THE natural anti-inflammatory breakfast.

Nothing comes out of a plastic tub at vast expense from a health store, in fact this is very economical. It goes like this:

The Ingredients for an Anti-Inflammatory Diet

I usually cut a pear, which are my favorite, into chunks and put it in the blender.

Depending on what is in the grocers it could also be an apple, papaya, mango, kiwi, grapefruit, pineapple or something that catches my eye.

Then I add half a cup of my seed mix made from equal parts of sunflower, sesame, flax and pumpkin. This delivers Essential Fatty Acids (Omega 3) and protein with all the goodies of the whole seed with its fiber. I buy a pound of each at a time. Mix them and store this in a big jar in the fridge.

Then I add berries. The dark berries, blueberries, blackberries and so on, are loaded with antioxidants called flavonoids and are just as good as the exotic, highly priced stuff from the Amazon. They freeze really well. My freezer is nearly full by the end of the season and this lasts the year.

This is the base. Then in go the super extras:

Tumeric is one of the very best anti-inflammatory herbs in nature. I can get fresh Turmeric in my local store, I put in a chunk about the size of the top joint of my thumb. This is a huge dose of curcumin with all the extras of the whole food.

I can also get fresh Burdock root, a wonderful liver and blood cleansing herb. A chunk the size of my finger goes in. This is called Gobo in Asia and eaten as a vegetable.

The Stinging nettle season is on where I live and I pick this from the wild.

They don't sting you when you blend them. The mix inactivates the sting and the natural minerals and anti-inflammatory action does you a power of good and suppresses allergies too. In goes a handful. They are great dried.

You can also cut up raw carrots or celery.

Here is the key: I put in all sorts of other things according to my mood and what's looking at me out of the cupboard.

The only limit is your imagination and your growing level of knowledge.

Play with it. You will save yourself hundreds of dollars in supplements and drugs.

Add water and blend until smooth, adding cold or warm water (almond milk unsweetened is also fine) as needed to achieve your preferred consistency. If you have more than you need for breakfast save some until later.

This mix, taken for breakfast or at any other time, is an excellent nutrient meal and a well-tolerated delivery system for large q uantities of nutrients and healing herbs.

Chapter 12 How To Jump Start The Anti-Inflammatory Diet

The anti-inflammatory diet has so many uses today it is surprising every one of the health, fitness and beauty gurus have not jumped on the simplest of diet changes and marketed them as the next big trend in weight loss, beauty and anti-aging. The fact is the anti-inflammatory diet can do everything other diets claim they can do and increase lifespan in the process.

So how do I jump start the anti-inflammatory diet?

Get a journal and write down all the foods you eat in a given week. Think of this first week as a natural eating time, so don't make any changes or eat anything you would not normally eat. Once the list is complete, head off to the Internet for a little research and education on the power of food over inflammation.

Many people are surprised by the effects seemingly healthy foods can have on overall body health and the prevention of illness. Sure, the market screams at the consumer about drinking more vitamin C and reducing calories, but what about the foods that seem healthy but really aren't? These foods will be found after a week of journaling before starting your anti-inflammatory diet.

Chances are, if these foods were purchased prepackaged; they will contain at least a small amount of trans fats.

Even the small, 100 calorie bites of cupcake marketed as healthy alternatives can contain up to 0.5 grams of trans fats. Eating just two of these little cakes a day for a week contributes a whopping 7 grams of trans fats - the only healthy level is 0 grams.

Did you eat a salad this week? Many people think eating a salad is a healthy alternative and it can be, without that fat laden dressing covering the healthy greens. One tablespoon of regular dressing can contain 100 calories and about 10 grams of fat.

The typical true serving is about ¼ cup per salad. That e q uates to 400 calories, 40 grams of fat and a -76 rating on the inflammation factor scale which measures the total inflammatory effect of foods on the body. The goal is to reach +50 or more.

Few people look at the foods they eat in an inflammatory way. But, the fact is that many common illnesses that can be life threatening is linked to inflammation. Choosing foods that contain no trans fats and low total fat is a healthy choice toward building your anti-inflammatory response. These changes are simple and anyone can jump onto the diet at any time.

The first steps, as with a lot of good diets are to begin to cut out the foods that are holding you back.

So if you regularly eat any of the above foods just mentioned then you need to start to cut them out. Eating these types of foods on an anti-inflammation diet completely defeats the purpose of what you are trying to do and will ruin your results.

Even if you don't suffer from inflammation but want to change your eating habits then following this type of diet will still be good for you. It will increase your health greatly and will help with fat loss.

The next steps would be to begin to introduce anti inflammation foods into your diet. Begin with adding the healthy omega 3 fats. Start to use extra virgin olive oil with your vegetables, coconut oil with your cooking, start snacking with nuts instead of chocolate bars and crisps and start to eat more fresh fish.

Supplementing with a high q uality fish oil supplement is also very important.

Hopefully you already eat a lot of fruit and vegetables in your diet, if not then you should start to add them now.

One of the great things about fruit and veg is variety.

There are literally hundreds of different varieties of fruit and vegetables available to us, all packed with goodness and FLAVOUR.

Drink green tea - Drinking green tea is proven to have anti- inflammatory benefits. Flavonoids in the tea have anti-inflammatory compounds which have been shown to reduce the risk of certain illnesses and diseases.

Beware that green tea contains caffeine.

Experiment with herbs and spices - Bring some life to your cooking and start to mix things up. Many people when cooking will add salt, sugar, mayonnaise and other easy options. Start to add garlic, ginger, turmeric, cayenne and other herbs and spices to give your meal some real flavour without sacrificing the healthiness of the meal.

Cut out foods that cause problems - If you find that you are intolerant to certain foods or you suffer from problems after eating certain foods then cut them out completely. Many people get bad reactions from wheat and gluten containing foods so try cutting out these foods and see if you notice a difference.

Chapter 13 How To Lose Weight And Feel Great With The Anti-Inflammatory Diet

The anti-inflammatory diet can make you feel great! "How," you ask. By cutting out or significantly reducing your consumption of pro- inflammatory foods. When these foods are cut from your diet, inflammation in the body reduces taking stress and strain from the joints and organs.

While following this diet your chance of weight loss also goes up. "How does this happen," by reducing your consumption of grain and wheat products, sodas, and other simple sugars that cause excess weight.

The fewer inflammatory foods we eat, the less inflammation we have in the body.

Grains, refined sugars, partial-hydrogenated oils, vegetable and seed oils are from modern man. These foods have been around a short time; hence, obesity and disease are on the rise. Humans are genetically adapted to eat fruits, veggies, nuts, lean meats, and fish, foods not related to chronic diseases.

Grains contain a protein called gluten. Gluten is the main cause of many digestive diseases, such as celiac disease, also contributor to frequent headaches.

They also have a sugar protein called lectins which has been shown to cause inflammation in the digestive system. Grains also contain phytic acid which is known to reduce the body's absorption of calcium, magnesium, iron, and zinc.

Lastly, grains contain high amounts of fatty acid biochemicals called omega-6 fatty acids which do cause inflammation. Fatty acid biochemicals known as omega-3 fatty acids are anti-inflammatory and found in fresh fish and green vegetables.

What Should I Eat? Anti-inflammatory foods

• All fruits and vegetables (raw or lightly cooked)

• Red and sweet potatoes

• Anti-inflammatory omega-3 eggs

• Raw nuts

• Spices such as ginger, turmeric, garlic

• Organic butter, coconut oil, extra virgin olive oil

• Fresh fish, avoid farm raised

• Meat, chicken, eggs from grass-fed animals

• Wild game such as deer, elk, etc.

• Water, organic green tea, red wine, stout beer

Chapter 14 How To Slow Down Cellular Aging With Anti Inflammatory Diet

Chemical oxidation of cells is a natural process for the body. However, these have some bad effects to the DNA and to electrons. When the cells undergo energy conversion process, the body produces harmful free radicals.

These free radicals are single electrons that follow a uni q ue path. When they meet paired electrons in your system, they snatch one of the paired electrons. This leads to cellular inflammation and DNA damage.

Cellular inflammation plays a huge role in the accelerated process of skin aging. Wrinkles appear faster and skin tissues become more fragile. Eventually, this leads to the loss of dermis elasticity. Thin skin condition and saggy dermis are just some of the problems you might have to deal with in the future.

One of the best ways to prevent cellular aging is to have an anti- inflammatory diet. Basically, foods rich in antioxidants are consumed. Antioxidants are molecules that fight harmful free radicals. These molecules also prevent the formation of free radicals.

Here are some tips on how to slow down cellular aging:

1. Instead of eating junk foods for your snack, eat dark colored berries instead. Blackberries, blueberries and raspberries contain a hefty amount of antioxidants that can fight cellular aging.

In addition to that, they are also rich sources of vitamins and minerals that can help fight the over-all skin aging process.

2. Always have vegetable side dishes for your main meals. Green leafy vegetables are rich sources of anti-oxidative molecules. They can further avoid cellular aging.

3. Increase your intake of cold water fish like Tuna and Salmon. They are the best sources of omega-3 fatty acids DHA and EPA. According to experts, nothing can prevent cellular inflammation more than omega-3 fatty acids. These fatty acids prevent inflammatory problems of any kind. This can even reduce joint inflammation so you can have better health.

A good diet is fundamental to young looking skin. But in addition to that, you also need to feed your skin with a natural moisturizer that contains beneficial ingredients like CynergyTK, Phytessence Wakame and Nano Lipobelle HEQ10.

CynergyTK is an ingredient found in the wool of sheep. This ingredient is made up of functional keratin, a complex type of protein needed for the production of collagen. Phytessence Wakame is a type of sea kelp that can prevent the sudden loss of hyaluronic acid.

This acid is essential for collagen lubrication. Nano Lipobelle HEQ10 is an antioxidant that can further avoid cellular inflammation. This has smaller molecular properties so it can easily penetrate the skin.

Chapter 15 The Anti-Inflammatory Diet For Arthritis Relief

Food and arthritis have a connection to each other and that is why changing your diet is one of the first pieces of advice an expert can give a person with inflammation in his or her joints. There are foods that can reduce inflammation and there are those that might worsen the inflammation.

A person with arthritis should follow the anti-inflammatory diet if he or she wants to get treated. To start an anti-inflammatory diet, one should know which foods he or she going to eliminate in one's diet and which foods will be added.

What are the foods that you should avoid and eliminate in your diet? When it comes to arthritis, it is always advised that the person affected should eliminate artificial foods like junk foods, those foods that have been processed and foods with added artificial flavorings and colorings.

A person with arthritis should also avoid meats that have high levels of fats and foods that are high in sugar. The reasons why these kinds of foods should be avoided by people with arthritis is that the saturated fats and trans fats found in these kinds of foods can worsen one's condition.

He or she should also avoid potatoes, eggplants and tomatoes because these are part of the nightshade family of plant that contains solanine that can provoke the pain.

Cutting these kinds of vegetables in people with arthritis have not been proven yet to be effective, but those who followed this kind of diet often show improvements with their condition and find relief from pain.

What are the foods to be added in your diet if you have arthritis? If you already know which kinds of foods you should eliminate in your anti-inflammatory diet, you should now know foods to add to your diet:

1.   Healthy fats and Oils: Fish oils are high in Omega-3 fatty acids that are essential to our health. This will help reduce the inflammation and prevent it from coming back. You will also get these fats in some seeds like flaxseed, pumpkin seeds, and sunflower seeds and also in Brazil nuts, almonds, cashew nuts and many more.

2.   Fruits and Vegetables: You should be eating more fruits and vegetables if you have arthritis because these have a lot of mineral, vitamins, antioxidants and photochemical that are beneficial for your arthritis and also to other conditions.

3.   Protein: Eating more proteins like fishes and other seafoods and poultry meats will also help people with arthritis.

4.   Drinks: You should need more li q uids to keep your joints lubricated. Drink more water, fruit juices, tea, vegetable juice with low sodium and non-fat milk.

Treating yourself for arthritis is not difficult if you know the kind of diet that is appropriate for your condition and if you know the foods to avoid with arthritis as well as the foods that must be eaten.

Chapter 16 Anti-Inflammatory Diet For Leaky Gut Disease

Leaky gut disease or leaky gut syndrome is a condition that can be caused by antibiotics, infections, parasites, toxins, or poor diet. The significant feature of the condition is alteration or damage to the bowel lining.

As the lining becomes more permeable than normal it allows microbes, undigested food, waste, toxins, or large macromolecules to enter. Some researchers believe that these substances have a direct effect on the body; others think the problem is an immune reaction to those substances.

Whatever has caused it for you, you probably just wish the symptoms -- everything from acne and indigestion to anxiety and fatigue to joint pain and constipation, to name a few - would go away.

Unfortunately, that wish can lead to treating just the symptoms. If you have Leaky Gut Disease, however, it's important that you don't just address the symptoms. You need to focus on the root causes of the condition.

One -- if not the main one -- of these root causes is diet. While practitioners disagree on a lot of things about Leaky Gut Disease (whether it even really exists, for example), the diet primarily recommended for those suffering from it - the anti-inflammatory diet - is generally acknowledged to be a healthy one for almost everyone.

The anti-inflammatory diet isn't really a diet; it's more of an eating plan. And if you do a little research, you'll find that there's not just one anti-inflammatory diet; there are several, each with a different spin. For our purposes here, I've tried to present what is a "generic" version.

This version does share with the others the concept that continued and out-of-control inflammation leads to illness and that following an eating plan that avoids inflaming the body promotes health and can help prevent disease.

In general an anti-inflammatory diet includes:

• Plenty of fruits and vegetables

• Plenty of whole grains (e.g., brown rice, bulgur wheat)

• Lean protein (e.g., chicken, fish)

• Anti-inflammatory spices (e.g., curry, ginger)

• Omega-3 fatty acids (such as those found in fish, fish oil supplements, and walnuts)

A reduction in

• Refined carbohydrates (e,g., pasta, white rice)

• Red meat and full-fat dairy foods

• Saturated and trans fats

- No refined or processed foods

Many who endorse this diet also urge that you avoid refined sugar and products that contain it as well as caffeine and alcohol. And

while drugs don't really fall into the diet category, have your doctor review your prescriptions and monitor your own use of OTC drugs, especially NSAIDS.

One word of caution regarding this plan: The effects you experience (i.e., an improvement in your symptoms) will not be as immediate as they would be if you treated yourself with medications.

You probably need to give the anti-inflammatory diet at least two weeks versus the hour or two a medicine might take. On the other side, this diet might have a bonus effect not usually found in medications: weight loss!

Chapter 17 Anti-Inflammatory Diet For Pain Relief

Most people are aware of mechanical causes of back pain such as ligament sprains, muscle, strains, slipped discs, etc. Fewer people are aware of inflammatory spinal pain, and the fact that our diets can lead to systemic inflammation those results in pain throughout the body.

It's important to be knowledgeable about the ways diet can promote inflammation, the foods that cause it, and a list of foods that actually fight inflammation.

There's no doubt that we don't make great food choices as a country, as evidenced by the ever increasing percentages of obesity and lifestyle diseases.

The standard American diet now depends largely on "comfort foods" where typically 60% of the calories come from oils, flour and sugar. While these foods taste good, they contain a high amount of arachidonic acid. Why should you care about arachidonic acid?

Arachidonic Acid

The two common fatty acids in our diet are Omega-6 and Omega-3 fatty acids. It is recommended that we consume a 1:1 ration of these fatty acids, but the average American diet can have as much as a 30:1 ratio.

When our diet is high in omega-6 fatty acids it shifts our tissue towards the pathogenesis of many diseases: proinflammatory, prothrombotic and proconstrictive.

One form of Omega-6 is arachidonic acid. While this acid in small   q uantities is essential for proper nutrition, in high q uantities it can promote excess inflammation throughout our bodies.

The arachidonic acid that we eat is eventually converted into prostaglandins that can cause pain and inflammation. To a certain extent, we are literally eating pain and inflammation with poor dieting.

Food High in Omega-6:Omega-3 ratio

In an effort to reduce inflammation, it is recommended that you avoid foods that have a high ratio of Omega-6 to Omega-3. The following is a list of some common foods that tend to have a high ratio.

Grains - 20:1

Seed and seed oils - 70:1 Soybean oil - 7:1 Chicken - 15:1

Potato Chips - 60:1

Benefits of Omega-3

The long-chain forms of Omega-3 fatty acids are DHA and EPA. DHA is the building block of brain tissue and EPA is its precursor. The following is a list of the benefits and conditions that are improved with Omega-3 acids in the diet.

• Healthier, stronger bones

• Improved mood regulation

• Reduced risk of Parkinson's

• Reduced risk of death from ALL causes

• Prevention of vascular complications from Type-II diabetes

• Gallstones

• Multiple Sclerosis

• Brain and eye development in babies

• Peripheral artery disease

• Preventing postpartum depression

• Combating cance

Foods High in Omega-3

• Flax seed oil

• Canola Oil

• Walnuts

- Fish

- Shellfish

- Krill

- Cod liver oil

- Omega-3 enriched eggs

- Pasture-raised meats

- Wild rice

- Beans

Anti-Inflammatory Foods

Along with focusing on foods that will provide the correct ratio of Omega-6 to Omega-3 fatty acids, there are also certain foods that have anti-inflammatory properties:

- Vegetables

- Fruit

- Sweet potatoes and other tubers

- Dark Chocolate

- Red wine

- Coffee and tea

- Ginger, turmeric, garlic and other spices

- Olive oil, Coconut oil and butter

A quality fish oil supplement needs to be in your diet. It's important to look for fish oil that has been molecularly distilled and contains at least 500mg of both DHA and EPA. There are plenty of fish oil supplements on the market that will advertise 1000mg of fish oil, but not all contain the recommended amount of those two acids.

Chapter 18 Tips For Practicing The Anti-Inflammatory Diet

Inflammation and aging go hand in hand as inflammation markers - especially the ESR (erythrocyte sedimentation rate) - slowly increase with each decade.

Many age-related diseases have inflammation as their common denominator and this is partially modulated by diet, so here are 10 easy tips to avoid the buildup of damaging inflammation products as much as possible:

Skip the sugar. Diabetes is the classical model of accelerated aging and sugar is made of empty calories anyway. The drive to consume glucose is innate, I know, but choose fresh fruit salads instead. You will get your sugar fix and some nutrients on the side.

The sweet tooth is the part most people find difficult about leading a healthy lifestyle and most traditional sweets are made of eggs, milk, butter and flour which are baked in the oven. That is the perfect recipe for advanced glycation end-products: you have proteins, sugar and high temperatures. The result is the Maillard reaction.

We already 'bake' from within as time passes by, so why add more glycation? You could try raw vegan desserts in exchange. These are made with nuts, seeds and fruits and don't involve any heating or baking, hence they are faster to make as well.

Lately, raw vegan cake shops have started to spring up everywhere. If there is no such place where you live, search online for raw vegan dessert recipes, especially if you have a weakness for sweets.

Don't let a day pass without eating a salad and add as many different fresh ingredients to it as possible.

Avoid smoked meat and cheese. Same for grilled meats. In both cases you have the unhappy mix of high temperatures and proteins which easily get denatured. The consumption of these types of products is linked to digestive cancers in populations where they are consumed in high q uantity.

There are better ways to prepare animal products, so why risk it? You could try marinated fish or non-smoked fermented cheese. Eat as few animal products as possible - once per week should be enough.

Use the lowest possible temperatures when cooking. If you are baking peppers, you could use a lower temperature and a longer time than if you would bake meat. Of course, you don't want to eat raw meats and get infections. Just use your best judgment when cooking.

Use high moisture levels when cooking. It's much better to boil and broil than to roast or fry ingredients. If you are a fan of crispy food, that would be difficult to implement.

On the other hand, there are many fresh vegetables and fruits that are naturally crispy if you feel the need for it - peppers anyone?

You don't need oil to cook. A ceramic pan/pot and a little bit of water will do and food will not stick. Cleaning is a breeze afterwards.

Avoid heating up fats. You can always add cheese, avocado, nuts and seeds in your recipes later on. Don't bake, fry or roast these.

Cheese will melt anyway if you place it over steamy fresh potatoes and the end result will be just as delicious.

Water should be your default beverage. Everything else - soups, teas, etc - is a bonus and they will never replace water, even if the human body will work with what is available and it will extract water from them.

People get more dehydrated with age anyway and many substances precipitate if you don't drink enough water, so why speed things up when water is so freely available and cheap? I guess if you are able to read this post, then access to clean water is not an issue. Unfortunately, that's not the case for everybody.

Eat as fresh as possible. If you want to eat meat or seafood, get it fresh and only use frozen ingredients if nothing else is available.

Don't cook more food than you eat in one sitting. Heated food is not as fresh or delicious as readily prepared one.

Too busy for that? I totally get it, that's why fresh vegetables, fruits and nuts were invented in the first place! You could add some quality yogurt and other healthy snacks when you don't have time to cook.

Chapter 19 30 Days Inflammatory Diet Meal Plan

Many people are surprised by the effects seemingly healthy foods can have on overall body health and the prevention of inflammation.

Few people look at the foods they eat in an inflammatory way. But, the fact is that many common illnesses that can be life threatening is linked to inflammation.

Choosing foods that contain no trans fats and low total fat is a healthy choice toward building your anti-inflammatory response. These changes are simple and anyone can jump onto the diet at any time.

The first steps, as with a lot of good diets are to begin to cut out the foods that are holding you back. So it is advisable to regularly eat any of the foods listed below. Eating these types of foods on an anti- inflammation diet completely helps in achieving the purpose of what you are trying to do and will boost your results.

DAY 1 to 7

Day 1- Coconut Pancakes   (Lunch)

Day 2- Blueberry Matcha Smoothie (Lunch)

Day 3- Pumpkin Pie Smoothi (Lunch)

Day 4- Leek And Spinach Frittata   (Dinner)

Day 5- Cherry Chia Oats   (Dinner)

Day 6- Banana Pancakes   (Breakfast)

Day 7- Fig Smoothie   (Lunch)

DAY 8-14

Day 8- Open Avocado Tuna Melts (Breakfast)

Day 9- Carrot Salad (Lunch)

Day 10- Chocolate Chili (Dinner)

Day 11- Mushroom Risotto   (Dinner)

Day 12- Mango And Avocado Salad (Breakfast)

Day 13- Kale Salad   (Breakfast)

Day 14- Spicy Ramen Soup   (Dinner)

DAY 15 – 21

Day 15- Miso Soup With Greens (Dinner)

Day 16-Chicken Chili (Breakfast)

Day 17- Lentil Stew (Dinner)

Day 18- Spiced Nuts   (Lunch)

Day 19- Blackberry Shrimp Salad   (Breakfast)

Day 20- Berry Freezer Pops (Lunch)

Day 21- Cauliflower Popcorn (Lunch)

DAY 22 – 30

Day 22- Cheesy Lemon Zucchini (Breakfast)

Day23- Chard Salad with Parmesan (Breakfast)

Day 24- Celery with Hummus (Dinner)

Day 25- Cauliflower-Mash (Faux Mashed Potatoes)
    (Dinner)

Day 26- Cacao Greek Yogurt with Strawberries(Lunch)

 Day 27- Brussels Sprouts with Black Bean Garlic Sauce
(Dinner)

Day 28- Asparagus Artichoke Salad (Breakfast)

DAY 29 – Oat porridge with berries. (Breakfast)

DAY 30 -Buckwheat and chia seed porridge (Dinner)

Chapter 20
Recipes

BREAKFAST RECIPES

1.   Coconut Pancakes

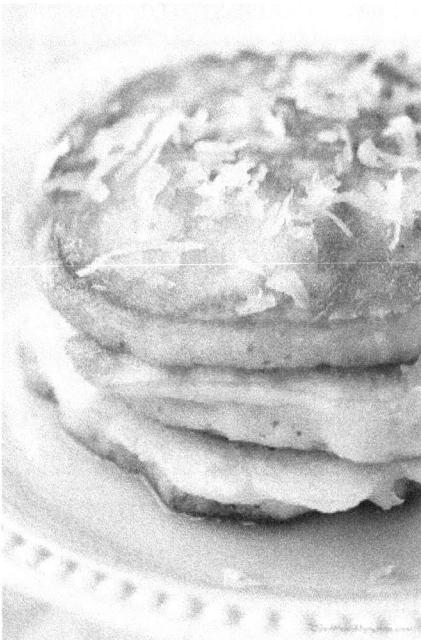

Ingredients

1   cup whole wheat pastry flour or whole wheat flour

2 tablespoons unsweetened shredded coconut 1 tablespoon sugar

2 teaspoons baking powder

¼ teaspoon salt

1 cup light coconut milk or 1 cup fresh coconut water from a mature coconut

1 egg

1 ½ tablespoons melted coconut oil or butter

Instructions

In a medium mixing bowl, mix together the dry ingredients (flour, shredded coconut, sugar, baking powder and salt).

In a separate bowl, whisk together the li q uid ingredients (coconut milk, egg and oil). If the coconut oil solidifies in contact with cold ingredients, let it warm up to room temperature for a few minutes, or microwave briefly in 30-second intervals until it melts and you can whisk it into the rest.

Pour the wet ingredients into the dry and stir until combined (a few lumps are ok). If you'll be using an electric skillet, heat it to 350 degrees Fahrenheit.

Otherwise, heat a heavy cast iron skillet or nonstick griddle over medium-low heat. You're ready to start cooking your pancakes once the surface of the pan is hot enough that a drop of water sizzles on contact.

If necessary, lightly oil the cooking surface with additional oil or cooking spray (I don't oil the surface of my non-stick griddle and my pancakes turned out great).

Using a ¼-cup measure, scoop the batter onto the warm skillet. Cook for 2 to 3 minutes until small bubbles form on the surface of the pancakes (you'll know it's ready to flip when about ½-inch of the perimeter is matte instead of glossy), and flip. Cook on the opposite sides for 1 to 2 minutes, or until lightly golden brown.

Repeat the process with the remaining batter, adding more oil as needed. You may need to adjust the heat up or down at this point. Serve the pancakes immediately or keep warm in a 200 degree Fahrenheit oven.

Nutrition Information

Calories 31.5, Total Fat 1.4 g, ,Cholesterol 37.2 mg, Sodium 114.3 mg, Potassium 35.0 mg, Total Carbohydrate 2.2 g, Dietary Fiber 1.0 g, Sugars 0.9 g, Protein 2.1 g

2.   Blueberry Matcha Smoothie

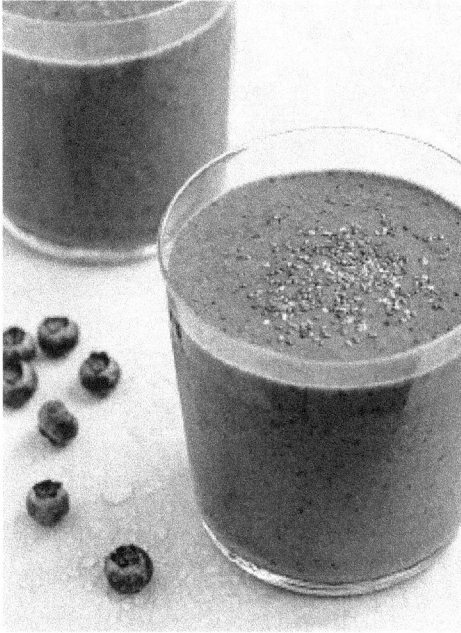

Ingredients

1 cup (155 grams) frozen blueberries

1 cup (30 grams) baby spinach

1 ripe banana

1 cup (240 ml) unsweetened almond milk 2 tablespoons old fashioned oats

1 teaspoon matcha powder I used ceremonial grade

Instructions

Combine all the ingredients in a blender and blend on high for 2-3 minutes, or until smooth and creamy.

Serve immediately, or store in the fridge for up to 2 days. Stir before serving.

Nutrition Information

Calories: 131, Fat: 2g, Sodium: 89mg, Carbohydrates: 28g, Fiber: 4g, Sugar: 14g, Protein: 3g

3. Pumpkin Pie Smoothie

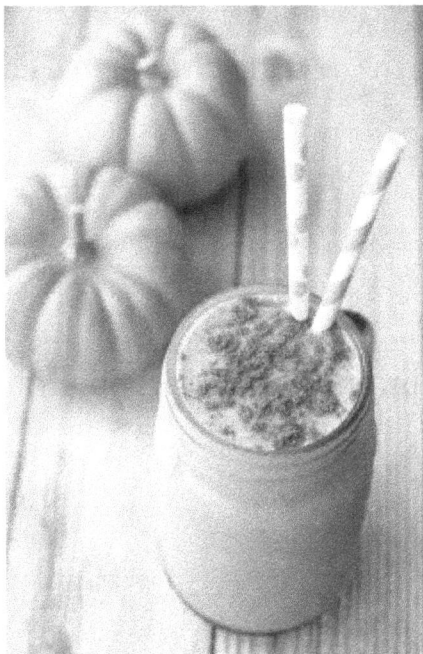

Ingredients

1/2 cup pure pumpkin puree 1 large banana

6-8 ice cubes

6 oz vanilla yogurt

1/2 tsp pumpkin pie spice

1 tsp agave nectar (or honey would work too), add more if you like it sweeter

3 Tbsp milk

pinch nutmeg and whipped cream, optional garnish

Instructions

In a blender (I love this one, it does a great job crushing the ice), combine pumpkin, banana, ice, yogurt, spice, agave nectar and milk. Pulse until smooth!

Pour into a glass and top with whipped cream and pinch of nutmeg. ENJOY!

Nutrition Information

Calories 261.3, Total Fat 1.0 g, Cholesterol 13.8 mg, Sodium 177.4 mg, Potassium 834.9 mg, Total Carbohydrate 51.8 g, Dietary Fiber

3.6 g, Sugars 21.5 g, Protein 13.2 g

4.   Leek And Spinach Frittata

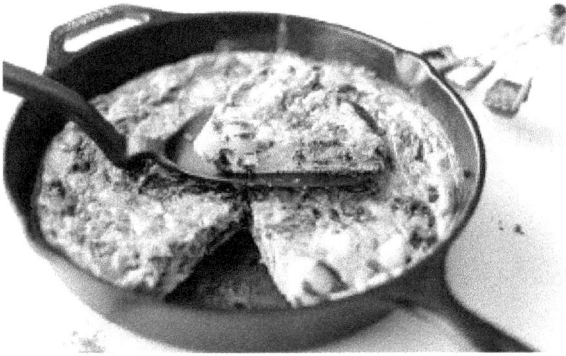

Ingredients

2 tablespoons unsalted butter

5 tablespoon extra-virgin olive oil, divided 1 cup cooked hash browns

1 large onion, peeled, cut in half and sliced thin 1 large leek, trimmed, rinsed well and sliced thin 8-10 free range brown eggs

3 tablespoons cream or whole milk 1/4 cup gruyere cheese

3 tablespoons parmesan cheese 1/2 cup baby spinach leaves

Salt and freshly ground black pepper to taste

1 cup cherry tomatoes

Instructions

Preheat oven to 350 degrees.

Combine eggs, cream and cheese in a medium bowl. Blend with a whisk or fork.

Heat 2 tablespoons oil in a medium ovenproof skillet over medium low heat.

Cook hash browns until they're golden and crispy. Remove from pan and set aside. Wipe pan clean.

Add the butter and 1 tablespoon oil to the pan.

Add the sliced onion to the pan. Reduce heat to low and cook slowly, stirring occasionally for about 15 minutes or until the onions turn golden brown and are lightly caramelized.

Add the leek and cook until tender and lightly browned for about 3 minutes.

Sprinkle the chopped spinach leaves in the pan.

Add egg mixture; stir gently to distribute spinach, onion and leek evenly.

Cover skillet and cook until eggs are partially set, about 5-6 minutes.

Uncover skillet, and bake for another 3-5 minutes or just until the center is set and the eggs are cooked through. Be careful not to overcook your frittata.

Remove from oven and loosen the frittata from the skillet. Cut into 8 wedges.

If using a cookie sheet:

Follow steps 1 - 7 then sprinkle the hash browns to the bottom of a cookie sheet.

Distribute the onion and leek mixture over the hash browns. Sprinkle the top with chopped spinach.

Pour the egg mixture over the top of the spinach.

Place the cookie sheet in oven and cook for 5-7 minutes or just until the center is set and the eggs are cooked through.

For the Pan Roasted Tomatoes

Heat 2 tablespoons olive oil to a pan.

Add the tomatoes and cook for over medium-low heat for about 1-2 minutes or until they begin to soften.

Nutrition Information

Calories 110, Calories from Fat 61, Total Fat 7.4g 12%, Cholesterol 172mg 58%, Sodium 215mg 9%, Total Carbohydrate 4.5g 2%, Dietary Fiber 1.1g 5%, Protein 6.8g 14%

5.   Cherry Chia Oats

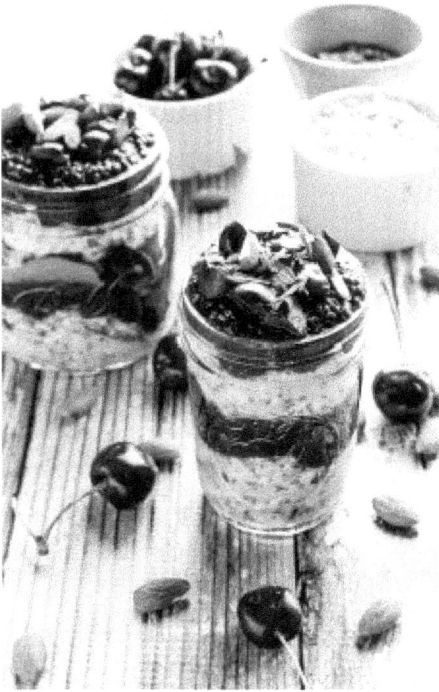

Ingredients

1/2 cup(s) Quaker Oats (quick or old fashioned, uncooked) 1 teaspoon(s) chia seeds

1 cup(s) frozen tart cherries

1/2 cup(s) cold unsweetened pomegranate juice

1/2 cup(s) nonfat milk or dairy alternative such as almond or soy

Instructions

Place oats and chia seeds in blender container. Blend until oats are finely ground. Add cherries, juice and milk. Blend until cherries are pureed and mixture is smooth.

For a smoothie bowl, substitute plain nonfat Greek yogurt for nonfat milk.

Nutrition Information

Calories 260.7, Total Fat 6.4 g, Cholesterol 5.7 mg, Sodium 96.8 mg, Potassium 86.3 mg, Total Carbohydrate 34.9 g, Dietary Fiber 6.7 g, Sugars 14.2 g, Protein 16.8 g

6.   Banana Pancakes

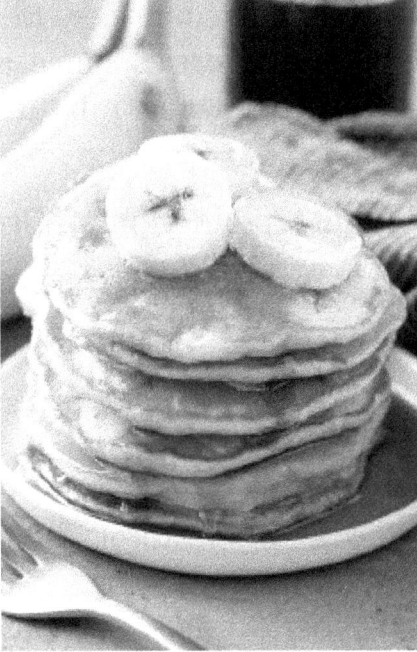

Ingredients

1 cup all-purpose flour

1   tablespoon white sugar

2   teaspoons baking powder 1/4 teaspoon salt

1 egg, beaten

1   cup milk

2   tablespoons vegetable oil

2 ripe bananas, mashed Add all ingredients to list

Directions

Combine flour, white sugar, baking powder and salt. In a separate bowl, mix together egg, milk, vegetable oil and bananas.

Stir flour mixture into banana mixture; batter will be slightly lumpy.

Heat a lightly oiled griddle or frying pan over medium high heat. Pour or scoop the batter onto the griddle, using approximately 1/4 cup for each pancake. Cook until pancakes are golden brown on both sides; serve hot.

Nutrition Information

193 calories; 6.6 g fat; 29.2 g carbohydrates; 5 g protein; 34 mg cholesterol; 246 mg sodium

7.   Fig Smoothie

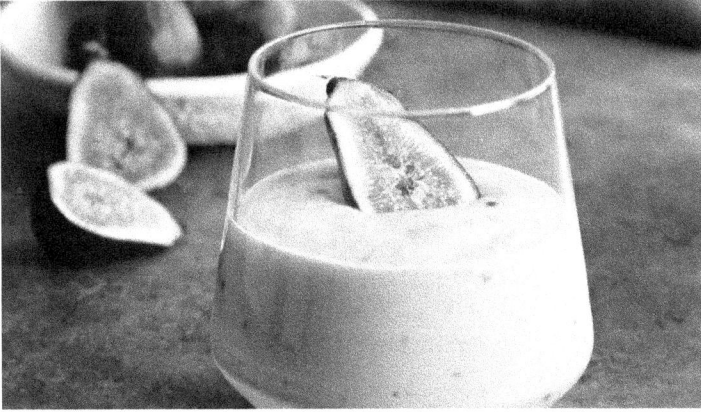

Ingredients

2 frozen bananas, peeled and chopped 6 fresh figs, halved

3/4 cup milk

3/4 cup orange juice

Directions

Place the bananas, figs, milk, and orange juice into a blender. Cover, and puree until smooth. Pour into glasses to serve.

Nutrition Information

Per Serving: 335 calories; 3 g fat; 77.7 g carbohydrates; 6.4 g protein; 7 mg cholesterol; 42 mg sodium

LUNCH RECIPES

1.   Open Avocado Tuna Melts

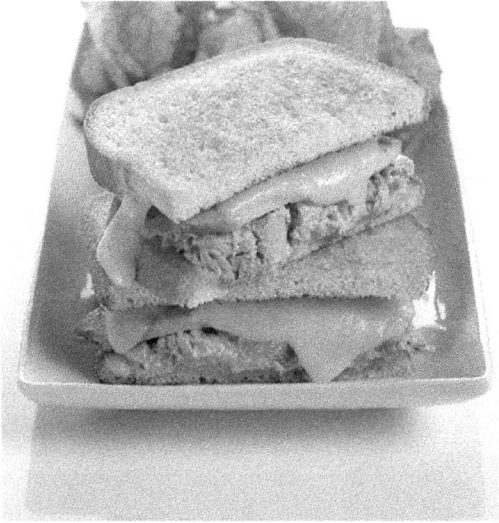

Ingredients

2 1/2 tablespoons olive oil

2 tablespoons thinly sliced shallots 1 tablespoon Dijon mustard

1/4 teaspoon black pepper 1/8 teaspoon salt

1 (6-ounce) can solid white tuna in water, drained and flaked

1 1/2 tablespoons fresh lemon juice 1 avocado

1   cup cherry tomatoes, quartered 1/3 cup shredded Swiss cheese

2   (6-ounce) pieces French bread, halved lengthwise and toasted

Instructions

Preheat broiler to high.

Combine first 6 ingredients in a medium bowl, stirring well to coat.

Place juice in a small bowl. Peel, seed, and chop avocado. Add avocado to juice; toss.

Add avocado mixture and tomatoes to tuna mixture; toss well to combine.

Sprinkle cheese evenly over cut sides of bread, and broil for 3 minutes or until cheese is bubbly.

Place 1 bread slice, cheese side up, on each of 4 plates, and divide tuna mixture evenly among bread slices.

SustainableChoice: Solid white tuna is albacore, the most sustainable choice among varieties of tuna

Nutrition Information

Calories 455 Fat 19.7g Protein 20.1g Carbohydrate 49.7g Fiber 5.3g Cholesterol 26mg Iron 3mg Sodium 860mg Calcium 140mg

2.   Carrot Salad

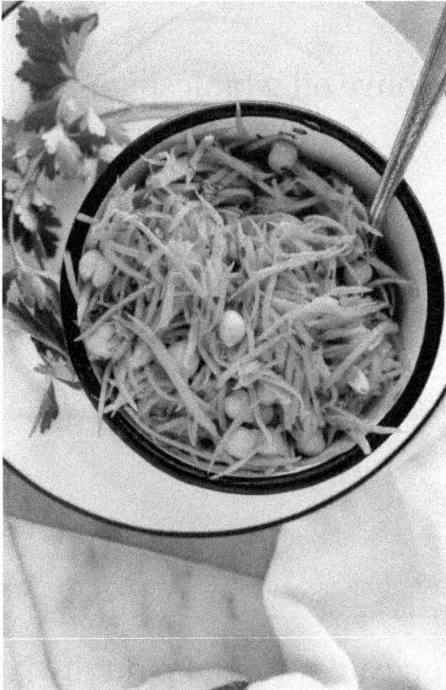

Ingredients

Carrot salad

1   pound carrots, peeled

2   tablespoons finely snipped chives or chopped green onion 2 tablespoons finely chopped fresh parsley

Optional: 1 can (15 ounces) chickpeas, rinsed and drained, or 1 ½ cups cooked chickpeas

Dressing

2 tablespoons extra-virgin olive oil 2 tablespoons lemon juice

2 teaspoons honey

1   teaspoon Dijon mustard

½ teaspoon ground cumin

¼ teaspoon fine sea salt

Instructions

To prepare the carrots: You can grate them on the large holes of a box grater, or use short strokes with a julienne peeler, or process them in a food processor fitted with a grating attachment. You'll end up with about 3 cups grated carrots.

Place the carrots in a medium serving bowl. Add the chives, parsley and optional chickpeas to the bowl.

To make the dressing, whisk all of the ingredients together in a small bowl until completely blended.

Pour the dressing over the carrot mixture and stir until the mixture is evenly coated in dressing. For best flavor, allow the salad to marinate for 20 minutes before serving. Toss again before serving. This salad keeps well in the refrigerator, covered, for about 4 days.

Nutrition Information

Calories 373 43%, Total Fat 28g gram 22%, Cholesterol 15mg milligrams 12%, Sodium 288mg milligrams 13%, Potassium 446mg milligrams 11%, Total Carbohydrates 32g grams 13%, Dietary Fiber 3.2g grams, Sugars 24g grams, Protein 1.8g

3.   Chocolate Chili

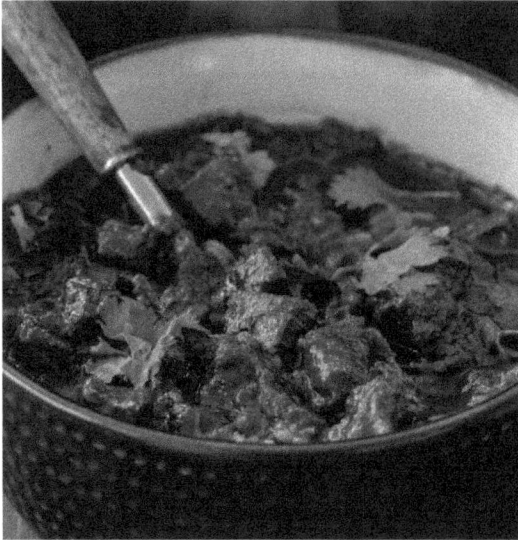

Ingredients

2   lbs ground beef 2 chopped onions

1 tablespoon plus 2 teaspoons chili powder

1   tablespoon ground cumin

2   tablespoons unsweetened cocoa powder 3 cloves minced garlic

2 seeded and minced jalapeño peppers

2 (15 oz) cans undrained ranch-style beans 1 teaspoon cayenne pepper

1   teaspoon dried oregano

2   (15 oz) cans drained and rinsed black beans

1   (15 oz) can diced tomatoes 4 cups tomato sauce

2   cups beef broth

Directions

In a large Dutch oven over medium-high heat, add the ground beef and cook for 2 minutes.

Next, add the onions, chili powder and cumin, and stir together.

Add the cocoa, garlic and jalapeños, mix together and cook for 2 minutes.

Next, add in the ranch-style beans, cayenne pepper and oregano, and cook for another minute.

Add the black beans, diced tomatoes, tomato sauce and broth, cover and simmer for 1 hour, stirring occasionally.

Garnish with sour cream, shredded cheese and chives if desired.

Nutrition Information

Calories 181.9, Total Fat 8.3 g, Cholesterol 31.6 mg, Sodium 227.9 mg, Potassium 508.7 mg, Total Carbohydrate 16.4 g, Dietary Fiber

6.2 g, Sugars 0.5 g, Protein 12.9 g

4.   Mushroom Risotto

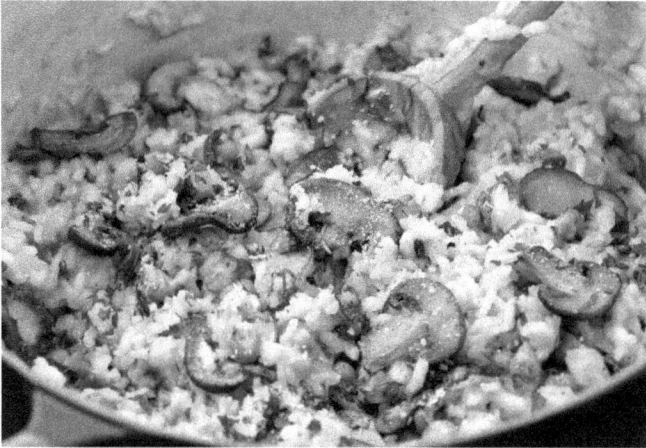

Ingredients

1 tbsp dried porcini mushrooms 2 tbsp olive oil

1   onion, chopped

2   garlic cloves, finely chopped 225g/8oz chestnut mushrooms, sliced 350g/12oz arborio rice

150ml/¼ pint dry white wine

1.2 litres/2 pints hot vegetable stock 2 tbsp chopped fresh parsley 25g/1oz butter

salt and freshly ground black pepper

freshly grated Parmesan (or similar vegetarian hard cheese), to serve

Instructions

Soak the porcini mushrooms in hot water for 10 minutes, then drain well.

Heat the oil in a large, heavy based saucepan and add the onion and garlic. Fry over a gentle heat for 2-3 minutes, until softened. Add the chestnut mushrooms and fry for a further 2-3 minutes, until browned.

Stir in the rice and coat in the oil. Pour in the wine and simmer, stirring, until the li q uid has been absorbed.

Add a ladleful of the stock and simmer, stirring again, until the li q uid has been absorbed. Continue adding the stock in this way, until all the liquid has been absorbed and the rice is plump and tender.

Roughly chop the soaked porcini mushrooms and stir into the risotto, along with the parsley, butter and salt and pepper. Serve with freshly grated Parmesan.

Nutrition Information

Calories 243, Total Fat 9.8g grams 19%, Cholesterol 16mg milligrams 11%, Sodium 268mg milligrams 12%, Potassium 426mg milligrams 10%, Total Carbohydrates 30g grams 4%, Dietary Fiber 0.9g grams, Sugars 3.8g grams, Protein 7.6g

5.   Mango And Avocado Salad

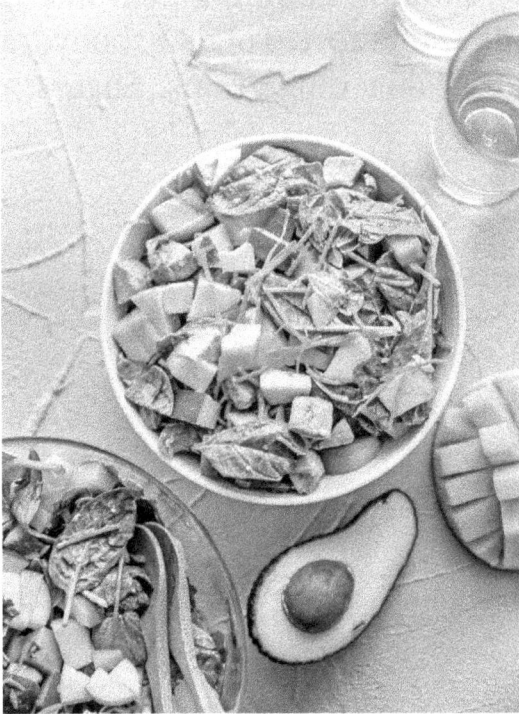

Ingredients

1   tablespoon balsamic vinegar 1 tablespoon lime juice

2   tablespoons extra-virgin olive oil 2 mangos, cubed

2 avocados, cubed

1/2 small red onion, diced

Salt and freshly ground black pepper

Directions

In a large serving bowl, whisk together vinegar, lime juice, salt and pepper to taste. Slowly whisk in oil. Toss in mangoes, avocado and red onion to coat. Serve immediately.

Nutrition Information

Calories 303.9, Total Fat 22.6 g, Cholesterol 0.0 mg, Sodium 10.5 mg, Potassium 599.9 mg, Total Carbohydrate 27.7 g, Dietary Fiber

8.4 g, Sugars 15.6 g, Protein 2.9 g

6.   Kale Salad

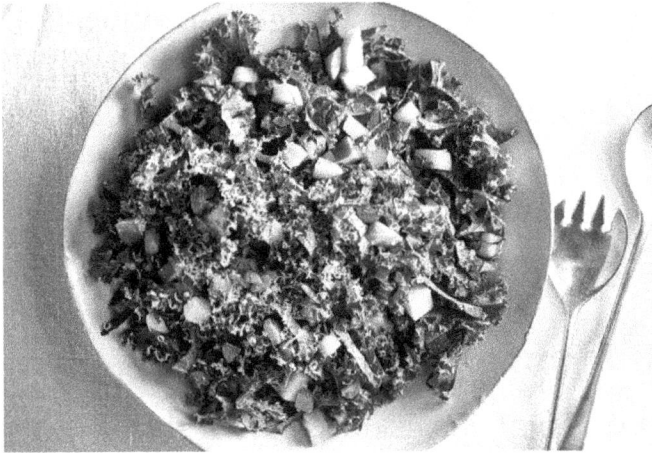

Ingredients

5 cups chopped kale 1-2 tsp olive oil

1/8 tsp salt

2 cups chopped broccoli 1/2 cup sliced almonds

1/2 cup cheese optional (cheddar or feta work great here!) 1/4-1/2 cup shredded carrots

 1/4 cup diced red onion 1/4 cup sunflower seeds 1/4 cup cranberries

Lemon Dressing 1/4 cup olive oil

2 tbsp fresh lemon juice

2 tbsp red wine vinegar 1 tbsp dijon mustard

1 clove garlic minced

1/2 tsp dried oregano 1/4 tsp salt

1/8 tsp ground black pepper

1   tsp honey or sugar adjust + add to taste

Instructions

First make your dressing by combining ingredients above in a lidded mason jar then shake well to emulsify. Dip a kale leaf in the dressing and adjust sweetener, salt, and pepper to taste. You can make this dressing as sweet or tart as your heart desires!

Next massage your chopped kale with a little olive oil and a pinch of salt. Rub with your fingers until leaves begin to darken and tenderize. This makes it taste great and gives the kale a silky texture!

In a large bowl, combine massaged kale, broccoli, almonds, cheese, carrots, onion, sunflower seeds, cranberries. Shake your dressing once more and pour about 1/3 of the dressing over the salad.

Toss to coat and add extra dressing, to taste.

Nutrition Information

Calories: 334, Fat: 26g, Saturated Fat: 3g, Sodium: 315mg, Potassium: 744mg, Carbohydrates: 19g, Fiber: 4g, Sugar: 4g, Protein: 9g, Vitamin A: 9985%, Vitamin C: 146.3%, Calcium: 192%, Iron: 2.7%

7. Spicy Ramen Soup

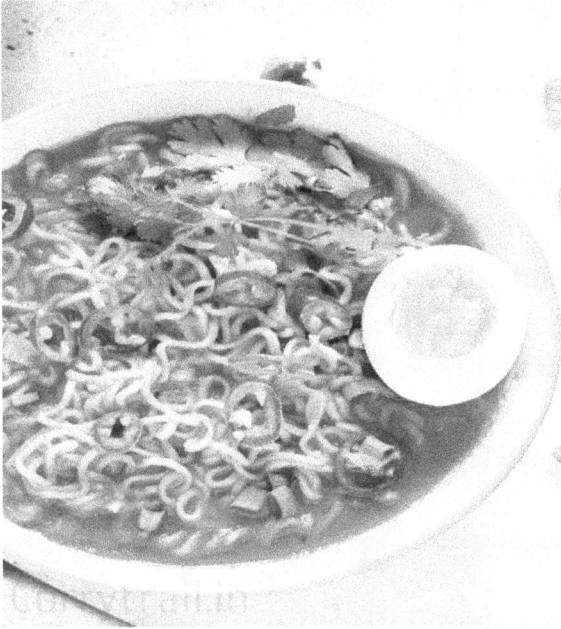

Ingredients

2   eggs

2 cups chicken broth see note #1 2 cup water

2 tbsp sriracha see note #2 2 cloves garlic minced

1   tsp fresh ginger minced 1 tbsp sesame oil

2   tbsp soy sauce

2 tbsp rice vinegar

10 oz white button mushrooms sliced 16 oz large shrimp about 20 shrimp

7 oz ramen noodles

1/2 cup scallions chopped 2 tbsp sesame seeds

Instructions

Place the eggs in a sauce pan and cover them with water. Bring to boil and once the water starts boiling, turn the heat off and put the lid on the sauce pan. Let the eggs sit undisturbed for six minutes.

After six minutes, run the eggs under cold water and peel them.

Set aside.

In a large pot, mix chicken broth, water, garlic, ginger, sriracha, sesame oil, soy sauce and rice vinegar.

Bring it to simmer, reduce the heat and simmer for about 25 minutes.

Add in sliced mushrooms and shrimps, cook for 2-3 minutes. Add in the noodles and cook for another 2-3 minutes.

Divide the spicy ramen between four bowls, top with half an egg, sesame seeds and scallions.

You can use vegetable broth instead of chicken broth.

Start with 2 tablespoons sriracha, this makes the ramen noodle soup pretty spicy. However, if you would like to have it even spicier, add some more sriracha right before serving.

If you would like to make this spicy ramen recipe vegetarian, swipe chicken broth for vegetable stock and use tofu or bokchoy instead of shrimp.

If you're going to have leftovers, make the noodles separately according to the instructions on the package and divide it between four bowls. Then fill the bowls with the soup base, shrimp and mushrooms.

Nutrition Information

Calories 290, Total Fat 11g grams 25%, Cholesterol 0mg milligrams 55%, Sodium 1310mg milligrams 13%, Total Carbohydrates 39g grams 8%, Dietary Fiber 2g grams, Sugars 3g grams, Protein 7g

8.   Miso Soup With Greens

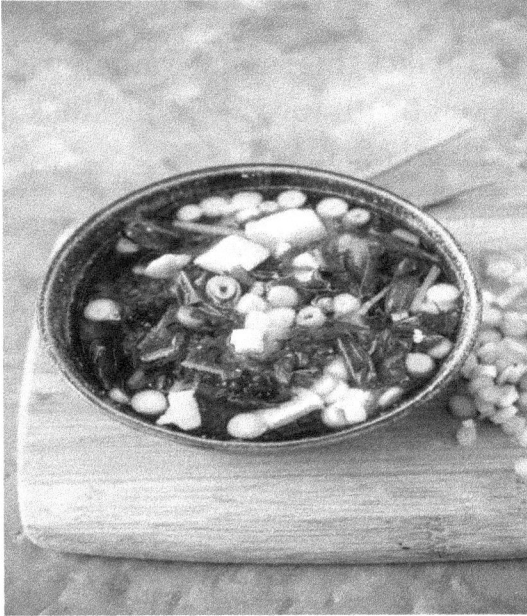

Ingredients

4 cups vegetable broth

1 sheet nori (dried seaweed // optional // cut into large rectangles

// 1 sheet yields 1/4 cup)

3-4 Tbsp white miso paste (fermented soy bean paste) with or without bonito (fish flavor, though bonito makes it non vegan- vegetarian-friendly)

1/2 cup chopped green chard or other sturdy green 1/2 cup chopped green onion

1/4 cup firm tofu (cubed)

Instructions

Place vegetable broth in a medium sauce pan and bring to a low simmer.

Add nori and simmer for 5-7 minutes.

In the meantime, place miso (starting with lesser end of range) into a small bowl, add a little hot water and whisk until smooth. This will ensure it doesn't clump. Set aside.

Add green chard, green onion, and tofu to the pot and cook for 5 minutes. Then remove from heat, add miso mixture, and stir to combine.

Taste and add more miso or a pinch of sea salt if desired. Serve warm. Best when fresh.

Nutrition Information

Calories: 170 Fat: 5g Saturated fat: 0.7g Sodium: 1817mg Potassium: 461mg Carbohydrates: 22.3g Fiber: 10g Sugar: 9g Protein: 13.6g

9.   Chicken Chili

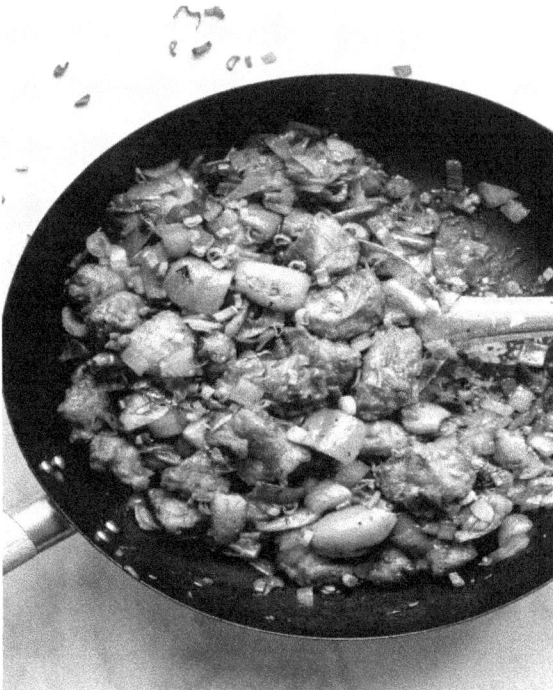

Ingredients

4 cups chopped yellow onions (3 onions) 1/8 cup good olive oil, plus extra for chicken 1/8 cup minced garlic (2 cloves)

2 red bell peppers, cored, seeded, and large-diced

2 yellow bell peppers, cored, seeded, and large-diced 1 teaspoon chili powder

1   teaspoon ground cumin

1/4 teaspoon dried red pepper flakes, or to taste 1/4 teaspoon cayenne pepper, or to taste

2   teaspoons kosher salt, plus more for chicken

2 (28-ounce) cans whole peeled plum tomatoes in puree, undrained 1/4 cup minced fresh basil leaves

4 split chicken breasts, bone in, skin on

Freshly ground black pepper For serving:

Chopped onions, corn chips, grated cheddar, sour cream

Directions

Cook the onions in the oil over medium-low heat for 10 to 15 minutes, until translucent.

Add the garlic and cook for 1 more minute.

Add the bell peppers, chili powder, cumin, red pepper flakes, cayenne, and salt. Cook for 1 minute.

Crush the tomatoes by hand or in batches in a food processor fitted with a steel blade (pulse 6 to 8 times).

Add to the pot with the basil. Bring to a boil, then reduce the heat and simmer, uncovered, for 30 minutes, stirring occasionally.

Preheat the oven to 350 degrees F.

Rub the chicken breasts with olive oil and place them on a baking sheet. Sprinkle generously with salt and pepper. Roast the chicken for 35 to 40 minutes, until just cooked. Let cool slightly.

Separate the meat from the bones and skin and cut it into 3/4-inch chunks. Add to the chili and simmer, uncovered, for another 20 minutes. Serve with the toppings, or refrigerate and reheat gently before serving.

Nutrition Information

Calories 226, Total Fat 8g 12%, Cholesterol 48mg 16%, Sodium 986mg 41%, Total Carbohydrate 19.68g 7%, Dietary Fiber 6.1g 24%, Sugars 5.7g, Protein 19.72g

10.   Lentil Stew

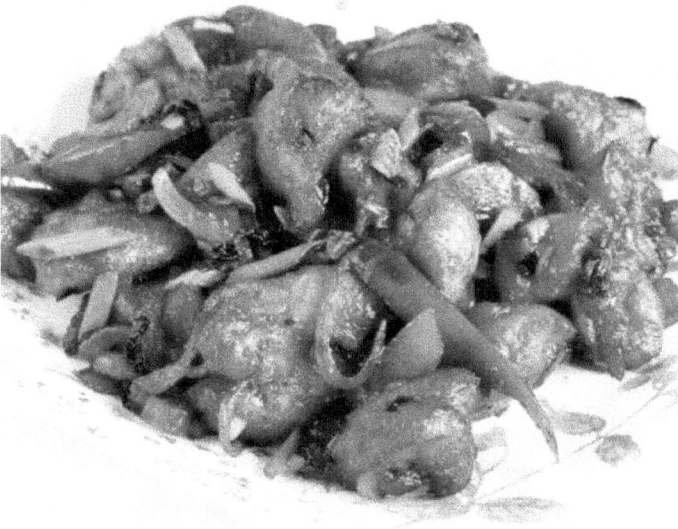

Chicken

Ingredients

4 tablespoons extra virgin olive oil 1 large onion, chopped

1   celery stalk, chopped

2   leeks, white and tender green parts, chopped 4 cloves garlic, minced

2 cups brown lentils

2 cups kale, chopped

1   large sweet potato, peeled and cut into large pieces
2 red potatoes, cut into large pieces

2   large carrots, peeled and cut into large pieces 1 15-ounce can chopped tomatoes

4 cups low-sodium vegetable broth 2 cups water

1 teaspoon cumin

1   teaspoon onion power 1/8 teaspoon cinnamon

salt and freshly ground black pepper to taste

Instructions

Heat the oil in a large pot or Dutch oven over medium heat.

Add the onions, celery, and leeks and cook for about 4 to 5 minutes.

Add the garlic and for another minute or two. Add the remaining ingredients

Bring to a boil, then cover, and let simmer on medium-low heat for

about 30 minutes or until lentils are tender.

Nutrition Information

Calories 241, Total Fat 1g grams1%, Cholesterol 0mg milligrams 21%, Sodium 503mg milligrams 29%, Potassium 1030mg milligrams 15%, Total Carbohydrates 45g grams 64%, Dietary Fiber 16g grams, Sugars 7.2g grams, Protein 16g

SNACKS RECIPES

1.   Spiced Nuts

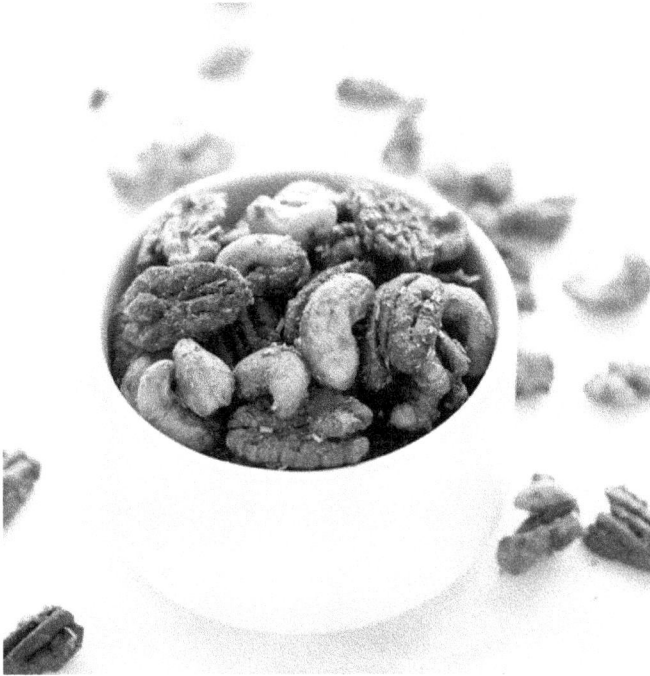

Ingredients

2/3 cup pecans (75 g), raw and unsalted 2/3 cup walnuts (75 g), raw and unsalted 2/3 cup cashews (95 g), raw and unsalted 2 tbsp maple syrup

1 tbsp oil of your choice (optional), I used melted coconut oil 1/2 tsp ground cumin

1/2 tsp salt

1/8 tsp ground black pepper

1/8 tsp cayenne pepper flakes 1 tsp dried rosemary

Instructions

Preheat the oven to 350°F or 180°C

Mix all the ingredients in a large mixing bowl (except the dried rosemary) until well combined.

Place the spiced nuts onto a baking sheet (lined with parchment paper or not, it's up to you) and bake for 20-25 minutes or until golden brown.

Remove from the oven, add the dried rosemary and stir until well mixed.

Serve warm immediately or keep in an airtight container at room temperature for 2-3 weeks. I prefer them cold.

Nutrition Information

Calories: 55, Sugar: 1.1 g, Sodium: 35 mg, Fat: 4.9 g, Saturated Fat:

0.9 g, Carbohydrates: 2.5 g, Fiber: 0.5 g, Protein: 1 g

2.   Blackberry Shrimp Salad

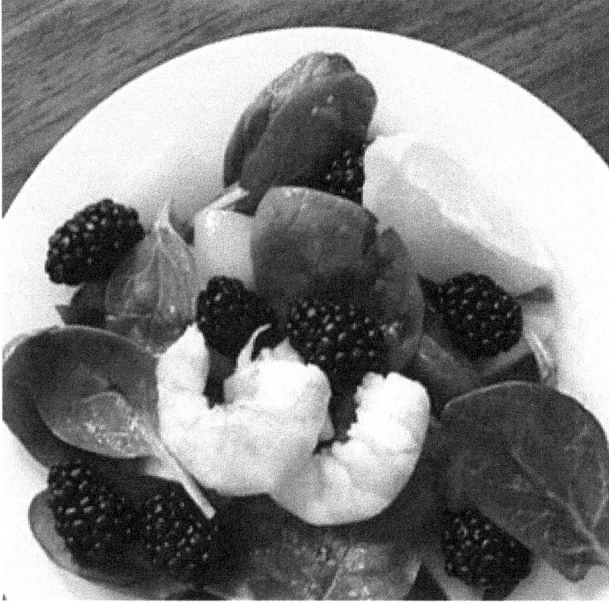

Ingredients

1/2 tsp Dr. Sears' Extra Virgin Olive Oil 2 tsp Lemon Juice

2   drops Agave Nectar 1/2 cup Baby Spinach

1/2 cup Yellow Bell Pepper (chopped)

1/2 cup Blackberries

2 medium Shrimp (cooked, chilled, chopped) Salt and Pepper (to taste)

Instructions

With a fork, whisk together olive oil, lemon juice and agave nectar to make the dressing.

Toss spinach and bell peppers with the dressing and transfer to a salad plate.

Top with blackberries and shrimp.

Nutrition Information

Calories 108, Total Fat 3g, Cholesterol 42mg, Sodium 229mg, Carbohydrates 14g, Fiber 6g, Sugar 4g, Protein 8g

3.   Berry Freezer Pops

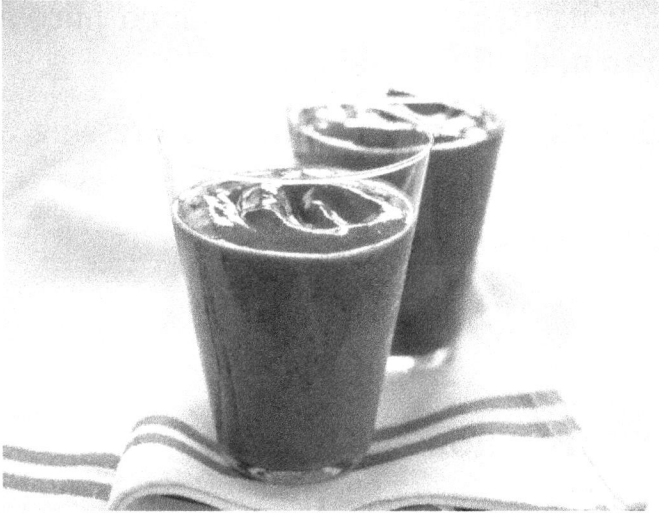

Ingredients

1 cup Strawberries 1 1/2 tbsp Almonds

3 cups Plain low fat yogurt - Stonyfield

Instructions

Put strawberries and almonds in a food processor and mix until very small pieces.

Add yogurt and pulse a few times.

Equally divide yogurt mixture in 6 small paper cups. Place a Popsicle stick in the middle of the yogurt.

Put in the freezer and freeze overnight.

Before eating, peel the paper cup.

Nutrition Information

Calories 93, Total Fat 3g, Carbohydrates 11g, Fiber 1g, Protein 7g

4.   Cauliflower Popcorn

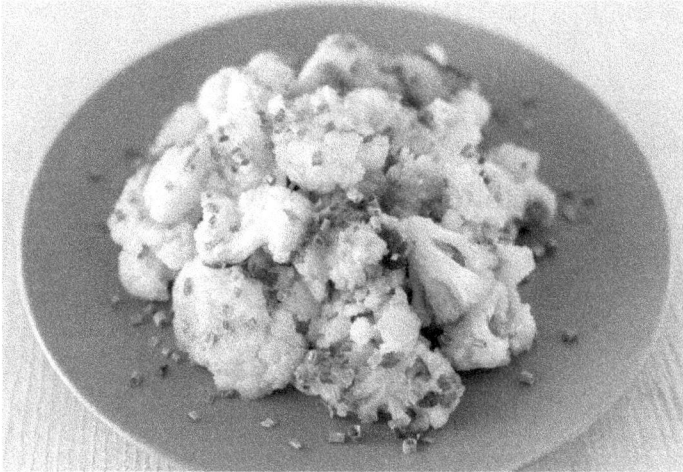

Ingredients

4 cups Cauliflower - cut into large florets 2 tsps Olive oil

Salt - To Taste

Instructions

Core and cut into florets.

Toss with olive oil to coat.

Sprinkle with a generous amount of salt or to taste.

Roast at 450°F until tender and browned, about 25-30 minutes. Serve with extra virgin olive oil for a drizzle.

Nutrition Information

Calories 90, Total Fat 5g, Carbohydrates 10g, Fiber 4g, Protein 4g

5. Cheesy Lemon Zucchini

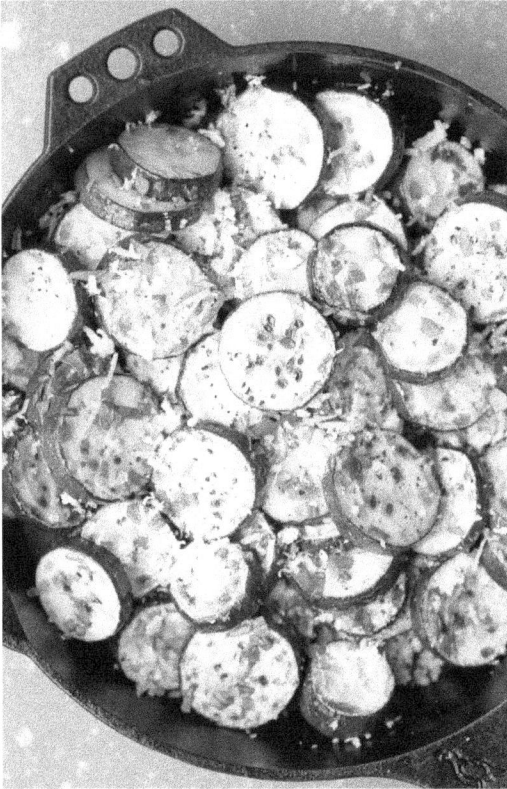

Ingredients

Cooking spray, olive oil Pam

Extra Virgin Olive Oil

3 lbs Zucchini, cubed

1/2 tsp Lemon zest

1/2 tsp Red pepper flakes

2 tbsps Kitchen Basics unsalted vegetable stock, or as needed Salt and pepper to taste

1/4 tsp Cayenne pepper - to taste 2 oz Fat-free cream cheese

2 tsps Dried oregano - or 2 tablespoons fresh, chopped

Instructions

Spray a skillet with cooking oil. Heat olive oil in skillet over high heat; stir in zucchini, lemon zest, and red pepper flakes.

Cook for about 2 minutes add stock as needed.

Stir in salt, black pepper, and cayenne pepper; cook and stir until zucchini is tender, about 5 minutes.

Stir cream cheese into zucchini mixture; cook until cream cheese begins to melt, about 1 minute.

Remove from heat and stir in oregano.

Nutrition Information

Calories 91, Total Fat 3g, Carbohydrates 13g, Fiber 4g, Protein 6g

6.   Chard Salad with Parmesan

Ingredients

1 lb Swiss Chard (remove stems, chopped) 3 tbsps Lemon Juice (freshly s q ueezed)

2 tsps Water

2 tsps Lemon Zest 1/4 tsp Salt

1/2 tsp Garlic Powder

1 1/2 tbsps Dr. Sears Extra Virgin Olive Oil 1/2 cup Parmesan (grated)

Pepper

Instructions

Remove stems from chard and finely chop, setting aside the leaves.

To make a dressing combine the lemon juice, water, lemon zest, 1/4 tsp salt and garlic powder in a small bowl. Slowly whisk in extra virgin olive oil. Set aside.

Put the chard stems and leaves into a large bowl and toss gently with the Parmesan and about 2/3 of the lemon dressing, serve the rest on the side.

Sprinkle with black pepper.

Nutrition Information

Calories 123, Total Fat 9g, Carbohydrates 7g, Fiber 2g Protein 6g

7.   Celery with Hummus

Ingredients

6 stalks Celery - halved lengthwise

1 oz Cooked skinless chicken breast - cut into small pieces 2 tbsps Hummus spread

3 tbsps Salsa

Instructions

Fill the well in the celery stalks with hummus and chunks of chicken.

If you prefer, cut the chicken into the hummus and use the celery like a spoon.

Nutrition Information

Calories 118, Total Fat 4g, Carbohydrates 13g, Fiber 6g, Protein 9g

8.   Cauliflower-Mash (Faux Mashed Potatoes)

Ingredients

1   16-oz bag Frozen cauliflower

2   tbsp Kitchen Basics unsalted chicken stock 3 1/2 tbsps 0% fat Greek yogurt

1 tsp Dr. Sears' Zone Extra Virgin Olive Oil, drizzle

Salt and Pepper - To Taste

Instructions

Cook cauliflower with the stock in microwave for 10 to 12 minutes or until cooked but still a bit crunchy, not mushy.

Put all ingredients, except extra virgin olive oil, into a blender, stick blender or food processor and puree until the consistency of mashed potatoes.

Serve and drizzle with extra virgin olive oil

Nutrition Information

Calories 89, Total Fat 3g, Carbohydrates 12g, Fiber 5g, Protein 7g

9. Cacao Greek Yogurt with Strawberries

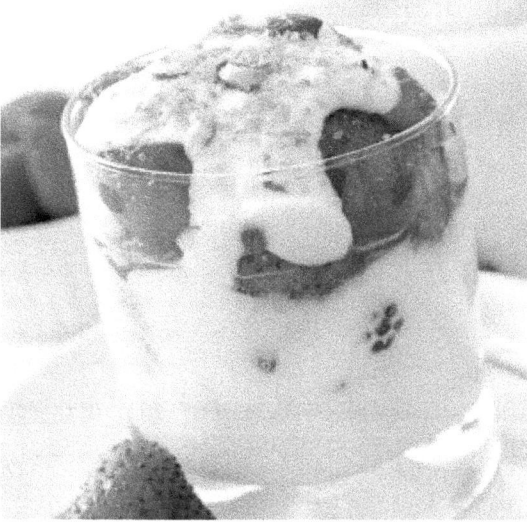

Ingredients

1/4 cup 0%-Fat Greek yogurt

1   1/2 tbsp Navitas Naturals Cacao Powder 1/4 cup Strawberries - sliced

2   tsps Almonds - sliced

Instructions

Stir the cacao powder into the Greek yogurt. Gently stir in the strawberries and almonds.

Nutrition Information

Calories 104, Total Fat 3g, Carbohydrates 11g, Fiber 4g, Protein 9g

10. Brussels Sprouts with Black Bean Garlic Sauce

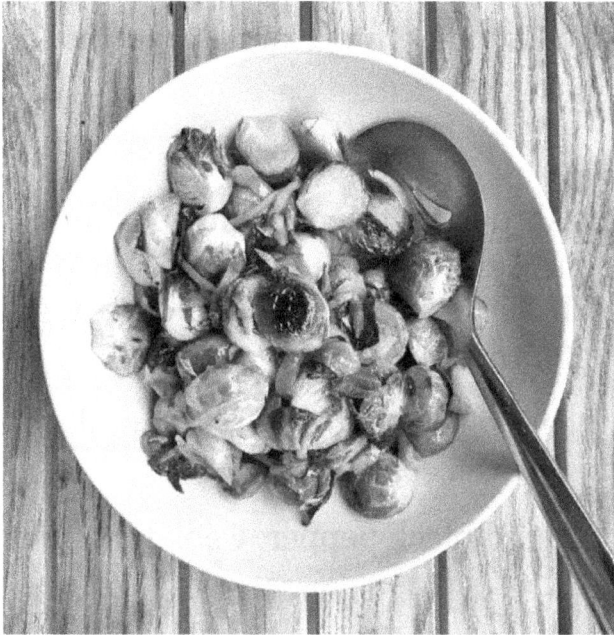

Ingredients

2 1/2 cups Frozen Brussels sprouts - thawed, q uartered
1 1/2 tsps Dr. Sears' Zone Extra Virgin Olive Oil

1/2 tsp Red pepper flakes

1 1/2 tbsps Black bean garlic sauce Ground black pepper

Instructions

Quarter the Brussels sprouts lengthwise.

Place the oil and chili flakes into a large skillet and place over medium-high heat.

Add the Brussels sprouts to the pan and cook for about 3-5 minutes or until the sprouts begin to brown a bit. They may absorb all the oil. If they do, just add a tablespoon of water or stock.

Add the black bean garlic sauce and stir until all the Brussels sprouts are well coated.

Add a pinch of ground black pepper. Cook for about 30 more seconds.

Take off heat and serve immediately.

Nutrition Information

Calories 112, Total Fat 4g, Carbohydrates 17g, Fiber 7g, Protein 7g

11.   Asparagus Artichoke Salad

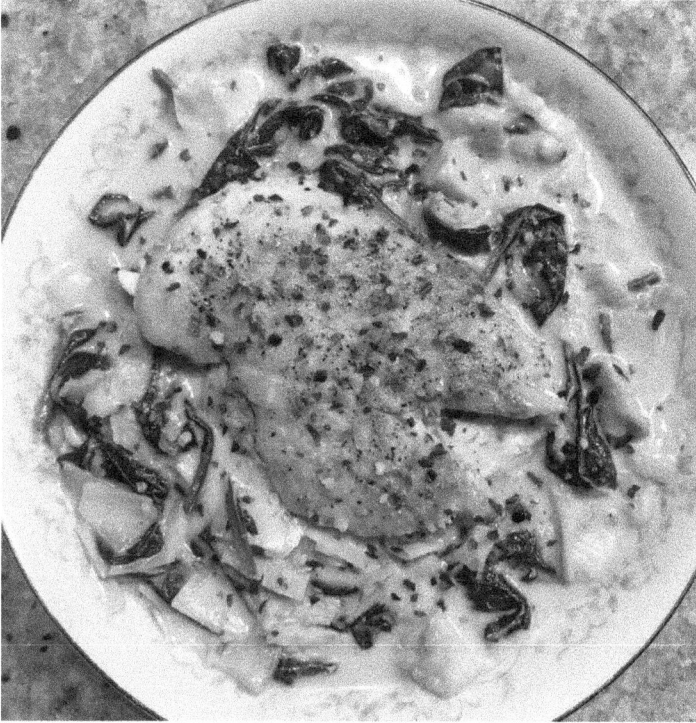

Ingredients

3 slices Red onion

3 tbsps Fresh s q ueezed lemon juice 1 1/4 pounds Asparagus

Salt and pepper - to taste

2 tsps Dr. Sears' Zone Extra Virgin Olive Oil 1 tsp Garlic powder

1 pint Cherry tomatoes - halved

1 (15-oz) can Artichoke hearts canned - quartered, rinsed

Instructions

In a large bowl soak the sliced onions in lemon juice. Set aside. Preheat the oven to 400°F.

Coat the asparagus spears with olive oil cooking spray and salt them well.

Place in a single layer in a foil-lined roasting pan and cook for 8- 10 minutes until lightly browned and fork tender.

Remove the asparagus from the oven and cut into bite-sized pieces.

Add the asparagus and all the remaining ingredients to the bowl with the onions and lemon juice. Mix to combine.

Serve chilled or at room temperature.

Nutrition Information

Calories 126, Total Fat 3g, Carbohydrates 23g, Fiber 13g, Protein 7g

Conclusion

There are many ways to stop the effect your diet has on inflammation. The easiest is adopting an anti-inflammation diet. Here are the three beginning steps to starting the diet off right.

Vegetables that offer a deep color are often better for your health. These deep colors often mean higher fiber content and better anti- inflammatory effects on the body. Herbs are also fantastic additions to an anti-inflammation diet. Here is a list of foods and herbs that will best help you to gain control over your inflammation.

When choosing seafood, the smaller the fish the better. Mercury is present in all fish and this is a compounding element. Eating the smaller fish like sardines, means eating from the lower end of the food chain with less mercury.

The idea is to boost healthy foods and eliminate unhealthy foods so for every good food you choose as part of your anti-inflammation diet, try taking out a processed food or fatty meat.

EFAs are present in nearly every food we eat, but the ratio of the different fatty acids is important as well as general consumption. Most people consume far more Omega 6s than Omega 3s and that can reduce the healthiness of even the best anti-inflammation diet.

Foods rich in Omega 3s include fish oil, olive oil, avocado, walnuts and grapeseed oil. An Omega 3 supplement can also be taken to boost this EFA in the diet. While flaxseed oil is the best source of Omega 3s, a fish oil supplement can also be chosen. It is important to make sure the fish oil is mercury free and tested for heavy metals.

Nuts and seeds are also perfect sources of EFAs. There is nothing hard about adding a handful of nuts or seeds to a salad or as a snack every day. For people with nut allergies, soy provides a healthy alternative. Soy is also a good source of lean protein which also has an anti-inflammation effect.

You may also hear about Omega 9 fatty acids. These are naturally occurring in the body, but that does not mean the amounts of this EFA when compared to Omega 3 and Omega 6 should not be taken into consideration. The effect of EFAs is heavily dependent on balance.

So far, stepping into an anti-inflammation diet has been really easy. During the elimination phase, however, some people have trouble giving up the foods they have grown to love the most. When listing the foods that need to be eliminated for their inflammatory effect on the body in order of importance, the list would include:

Trans fats are present in hydrogenated oils like margarine. Despite many labels ready "0 trans fats"; they are still in those products in small amounts. Sugar is just not good for the body. Replacing processed sugar with natural cane may be a healthier alternative.

Refined carbohydrates include processed flour which is used in nearly every loaf of bread and baked goods sold in a package. Try baking for yourself with whole grain flour instead.

Food allergens often include gluten, soy, eggs, dairy and nuts. These foods will increase inflammation in the body immediately if there is a food allergy. Medical food allergy testing can provide a specific list of food that will cause a reaction in the body.

If you want to find out which foods you are allergic to on your own, keep a journal and eliminate the foods one by one for a few days. Then, eat the food in q uestion to see if there is a change or reaction. Mild food allergies often affect gastrointestinal systems with constipation or diarrhea. Rashes and hives, both inflammatory responses, may also appear.

www.ingramcontent.com/pod-product-compliance
Lightning Source LLC
Chambersburg PA
CBHW050724030426
42336CB00012B/1403